Hormone Replacement Therapy

Hormone
Replacement
Therapy

Conventional Medicines and Natural Alternatives, Your Guide to Menopausal Health Care Choices

Updated Edition

Linda Laucella

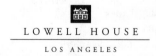

LOWELL HOUSE

LOS ANGELES

CONTEMPORARY BOOKS

CHICAGO

Library of Congress Cataloging-in-Publication Data

Laucella, Linda.
    Hormone replacement therapy: your personal guide to making the
right decisions / Linda Laucella.
        p. cm.
    Includes bibliographical references and index.
    ISBN 1-56565-343-2
            1-56565-154-5 (paperback)
            1-56565-805-1 (updated edition)
    1. Menopause—Hormone therapy—Popular works. 2. Menopause—
Hormone therapy—Miscellanea. I. Title.
RG186.L38 1994
6118.1'75061—dc20

                                                    94-30125
                                                    CIP

Requests for such permissions should be addressed to:

Lowell House
2020 Avenue of the Stars, Suite 300
Los Angeles, CA 90067

Publisher: Jack Artenstein
Associate Publisher, Lowell House Adult: Bud Sperry
Director of Publishing Services: Rena Copperman
Managing Editor: Maria Magallanes
Text Design: Janice Jenkins

Manufactured in the United States of America
10 9 8 7 6 5 4 3 2 1

Contents

Introduction

Facing menopause and deciding whether to choose hormone replacement therapy can be a complicated and bewildering experience for a woman. Although hormone replacement started out by using estrogen alone, now it includes different kinds of estrogen, progestins, natural progesterone, and testosterone in various combinations and dosages. Each hormone offers different health benefits and some are known to have health risks and side effects. Because of the side effects and health risks experienced by some women taking *HRT*, many of them are trying to make decisions about continuing it.

How can this book help you make decisions about *HRT* and its benefits for your overall health? This guide combines the knowledge of experts from various aspects of women's health in order to explain what happens to your body during and after menopause, and suggests what *HRT* and natural healthcare choices you can make. Because I am not a healthcare professional, no preferred treatment program or medical point of view is expressed. I am a healthcare consumer just as you are, looking for the most effective care I can find to maintain my current good health into the later years of life. The main difference between you and me is that I am a writer who knows where to find the information about women's healthcare that you would like to know.

Let's begin by putting menopause into perspective: Menopause is not a disease that needs to be treated, although your hormonal changes during menopause can result in serious health problems later in life. It does not signal the end of your vitality, your sexuality, or your womanhood. Menopause is only one of a natural series of changes we women undergo throughout our lives. Our first dramatic change of life was when we entered adulthood during puberty. Beginning at that time we become aware of the constant ebb and flow of hormones within our bodies. Since then we have learned to anticipate the complex series of pain and pleasure that result from living in a woman's body. During our late thirties to mid-fifties our ovaries slow down their production of hormones, we enter our second dramatic change of life, and we need to understand that our bodies will operate differently.

Although the cessation of hormone production is gradual, the effects on our bodies are obvious to us. Not only do we feel different, we begin to look different as well. Of course that can make us fearful. Our first change of life, during puberty, was considered good. Despite the physical discomfort and emotional confusion we felt when our ovaries began to produce hormones, we were rewarded with the enhanced physical appearance of becoming a woman and the ability to produce children. But this second change of life called menopause is perceived differently. At times it can feel very mysterious and confusing to us.

While preparing to work on this book, I asked myself, how women can view this phase of life realistically, approaching it and living through it without fear. I believe knowledge and preparation are the keys that open the door, inviting us all to enter our middle and later years of life more in control than ever of our bodies, our emotions, and our lives.

Many women experience a new calmness after their body releases the intensity of its monthly hormone cycles. These women suggest that the menopausal transition is a time to listen to your body, to hear what it is telling you, accept the changes it is making, and embrace the new person you are becoming.

After our bodies complete menopause, we are free to enjoy sexual intercourse without fear of pregnancy. But then our pelvic organs begin to change because they are no longer stimulated by estrogen. At the same time our appearance begins to change, and we fear no longer feeling attractive and desirable because we have heard that our youthful feminine appearance is largely controlled by our hormones.

Hormone replacement therapy seems like the instant answer, a woman's fountain of youth, by boosting the hormone levels in our bodies and stopping the aging clock. But it isn't that simple. Although *HRT* can benefit a woman's appearance in some ways, it does not stop the natural aging process, and it can have side effects. The seriousness of the side effects depends on a woman's own individual health profile.

Today, experts believe the risks of developing breast or uterine cancer, heart disease, and osteoporosis can be traced through your family history. The risks can also be affected by your age, diet, lifestyle, and the kind of replacement hormones you take.

A large percentage of women in America pass through menopause into later life with ease, in comfort, and are able to maintain their good health. Women in other cultures breeze through menopause with no adverse effects. We can learn a lot from these women and integrate their secrets into our own lives. By regulating the hormone balance within our bodies, our good health and radiant appearance can be maintained and enhanced. As a result, our sense of self-confidence and stability will enable us to maintain inner peace. Then we can handle whatever discomfort and distress menopause may bring to us because we'll feel good enough physically and emotionally to continue living the full, useful lives we have created for ourselves.

How can you regulate the hormone balance within your body to offset the discomforts of menopause as your ovaries are gradually producing less hormones? Conventional medicine often prescribes *HRT* and suggests accompanying dietary and lifestyle changes. That program works for many women. Other women prefer more natural hormones, programs, and remedies that may include nutritional supplements, herbs, or acupuncture, with the guidance of alternative healthcare professionals, along with dietary and lifestyle changes. Many women combine elements of these various approaches. Every woman is unique.

How do you decide what is right for you? First, learn as much as you can about your own body and about the healthcare options available to you. Talk with healthcare professionals you trust, those who really listen to you and seem genuinely interested in your well-being. Talk with other women about their experiences and yours. Read about menopause and women's healthcare. Write down what you know, learn, and feel about menopause. Do not limit yourself to a single point of view or program based on the advice of anyone, whether it's from a healthcare professional or from a friend. This decision is yours alone to make.

What if you try something and it doesn't seem to be working right away? After making informed healthcare choices based on what feels right to you and embarking on a healthcare program, give it a reasonable period of time before deciding it's not effective. Even though you have a right to change your mind as often as you choose, your body may need time to catch up with your mind. The hormonal system of your body is complicated; constant, sudden changes will only confuse it. This is a time to be gentle with your body—and with yourself.

While reading this book, you will find that some information is repeated from one chapter to the next. This is done deliberately to present as complete a picture as possible in each chapter so you can be well informed on the choices available. Suggested dosages of hormones, vitamin/mineral supplements, herbs, or other natural remedies are generally not included because they must be adjusted to each woman's individual needs by a healthcare professional. The Suggested Reading List and Resources at the back of the book will guide you to more information if you need it.

Now, more than ever, the independent mind of the mature

woman recognizes that the ultimate responsibility for her own emotional and physical well-being is hers alone. Women have become seekers. We gather information, we weigh what we have learned and, finally, we seek to apply that knowledge within our own lives.

This book was written in that spirit of the modern woman. It does not take a position. It does not presume to tell a woman what is best for her. It presents the facts and suggests what your options might be by answering the questions many women are asking about hormone replacement therapy and its alternatives.

CHAPTER 1
▲ ▲ ▲

What Happens to a Woman's Body During and After Menopause?

Many women approach their menopausal years with limited information about how their bodies function and what changes they can anticipate. By better understanding your own body, you will be prepared to make the menopausal transition and decisions about your healthcare without fear and confusion.

WHAT IS MENOPAUSE?

Strictly speaking, menopause occurs when a woman stops having menstrual periods. However, menopause is generally referred to as the transition period every woman goes through naturally, usually during the middle years of life. At that time the production of hormones by the ovaries becomes erratic and eventually stops.

DOES MENOPAUSE HAPPEN ALL AT ONCE OR IS IT GRADUAL?

The average woman's ovaries begin to gradually produce lower levels of hormones during her thirties. This decline may continue to be gradual or it may become erratic during her forties, resulting in irregular menstrual periods. Most women are not aware of the change in hormone production within their bodies until their menstrual periods become irregular or stop. At that time, the

1

ovaries may still be producing hormones, but not enough to maintain the reproductive qualities of the uterus and eventually the menstrual periods stop altogether.

When a woman's ovaries are surgically removed before she reaches natural menopause, she will go through menopause immediately.

HOW DOES A WOMAN KNOW WHEN SHE'S GOING THROUGH MENOPAUSE?

The first signs of menopause are usually irregular menstrual periods, possibly accompanied by hot flashes, night sweats, and a lack of energy. However, some women experience hot flashes and night sweats while their menstrual periods are still regular.

Menstrual irregularity, hot flashes, and night sweats before menopausal age may be a warning that abnormal hormone production is a symptom of a serious health condition involving the ovaries, uterus, or endocrine system, therefore, immediate attention by a physician is recommended.

CAN A DOCTOR TELL IF YOU'RE DEFINITELY EXPERIENCING MENOPAUSE?

A physician can check your blood hormone levels to determine if you are experiencing menopausal hormone irregularity. However, blood hormone levels in many women become erratic during the menopausal transition, so they could indicate menopause one week and be normal the next.

This a time to report to your doctor any other discomforts or symptoms of abnormal health conditions, especially heart palpitations or bone discomfort. As we will discuss later in this chapter and in other chapters of this book, many of the signs associated with menopause can also be indications that you need additional medical evaluations to insure that they are not symptoms of more serious health conditions.

DO MOST WOMEN CONSULT A PHYSICIAN WHEN THEIR MENSTRUAL PERIODS BECOME IRREGULAR OR STOP?

Women often consult a physician when their menstrual periods stop in order to confirm whether or not they are pregnant. Others may be experiencing other discomforts associated with menopause and want to make sure their symptoms do not indicate a serious health problem.

WHY DO A WOMAN'S MENSTRUAL CYCLES BECOME IRREGULAR DURING THE MENOPAUSAL TRANSITION?

Not all women experience irregular menstrual cycles during the menopausal transition, however it is common and usually is caused by decreased or irregular hormone production by the ovaries.

Estrogen is produced in the ovaries by ripening egg follicles. Estrogen production stimulates the uterus, causing the uterine lining to build up. After a mature egg is released by the ovaries (ovulation), progesterone production begins. Progesterone prepares the uterine lining to be implanted with a fertilized egg, resulting in pregnancy. If a fertilized egg does not implant in the uterus, progesterone levels drop off dramatically, triggering the uterus to shed its lining (menstrual period).

In a healthy woman, irregular menstrual periods usually indicate lower levels of hormone production by her ovaries. Menstrual periods stop entirely when a woman's ovaries stop producing hormones.

DOES MENSTRUATION CONTINUE AS LONG AS A WOMAN IS OVULATING?

Ovulation stops when the ovaries have run out of eggs to ripen or when the remaining eggs are too old. That results in a loss of estrogen and progesterone production and the menstrual periods stop.

DO THE OVARIES STILL PRODUCE ESTROGEN AFTER PROGESTERONE PRODUCTION STOPS?

Studies indicate most women stop producing progesterone first.

Estrogen production by the ovaries and uterus continues to a degree until some time after menopause when it finally stops.

DOES A WOMAN'S BODY STOP PRODUCING ESTROGEN ALTOGETHER AFTER MENOPAUSE?

After the ovaries stop producing estrogen, the adrenal glands take over, producing a weaker form of estrogen (estrone) and the body continues to convert androgens (male hormones) from body fat into estrogen.

WHAT EFFECTS DO THESE WEAKER FORMS OF ESTROGEN HAVE ON A WOMAN'S BODY?

Although the estrogen produced by the adrenal glands and con- verted from body fat is a much less potent form of estrogen than is produced by the ovaries, it can help alleviate some common discomforts associated with menopause, such as hot flashes, sweating, inability to sleep, and vaginal dryness. A woman with healthy adrenal glands usually experiences an easier menopause with less physical discomfort.

Whether or not weaker estrogen production will prevent a woman from developing pelvic organ atrophy, osteoporosis, or heart disease after menopause depends on her overall health, diet, and lifestyle factors. These factors may also influence a woman's decisions about taking replacement hormones.

IF ESTROGEN IS CONVERTED BY THE BODY FROM FAT, DO HEAVIER WOMEN HAVE MORE ESTROGEN THAN THIN WOMEN?

Heavier women usually do have higher estrogen levels than thin women during menopause. For that reason heavier women may have a smoother transition through menopause. Very thin women often experience menopause earlier in life.

IS IT BETTER TO BE HEAVIER WHEN ENTERING MENOPAUSE?

The estrogen converted by the body from fat may be strong enough to alleviate many of the discomforts associated with menopause, assisting to some degree in preventing pelvic organ atrophy, osteoporosis, and heart disease. However, it is well known that too much body fat is detrimental to the overall health of a woman in many ways. Entering menopause at an appropriate weight for your own body type and maintaining that weight through adequate nutritional intake and exercise is best for a woman's overall health.

BESIDES SEEING A DOCTOR, HOW DOES A WOMAN KNOW WHEN HER BODY HAS STARTED THE MENOPAUSAL TRANSITION?

Generally, there are three stages of menopause. During the period of time known as perimenopause, early signs of menopause usually include physical discomforts but not serious health conditions.

Once a woman's menstrual periods have stopped she has reached menopause and may then be faced with health conditions that, while not life threatening, can lead to later health problems.

Finally, after a woman's body has made the hormonal adjustments, she faces postmenopausal changes in her body that may require serious attention in order for her to maintain optimal health into her later years of life.

WHAT ARE THE EARLY SIGNS OF MENOPAUSE?

Perimenopause signs may include:

- Irregular menstrual periods; during perimenopause a woman's menstrual periods usually change. Sometimes menstrual cycles become shorter and diminish, sometimes they become longer with increased flow. Some women's periods just stop one day and never resume. The menstrual period may also begin to be accompanied by cramping and clotted blood flow.

- Hot flashes may occur initially at night, and then during the day, especially after eating or physical activity. Hot flashes seem to occur most often before the onset of a menstrual period and are sometimes stronger when the period is delayed. Hot flashes may also be accompanied by sweating and heart palpitations as well as leg cramping at night.

- Sleep disturbances are usually caused by hot flashes, night sweating, and leg cramping.

- Emotional changes or sudden changes of temperament may include fatigue, depression, anxiety, mood swings, irritability, aggression, insomnia, even compulsive eating.

- Disorders of the reproductive organs, such as uterine fibroids and ovarian cysts, may be discovered during a physical examination.

- Vaginal secretions may increase or decrease.

WHAT CAUSES THESE EARLY SIGNS OF MENOPAUSE?

The body is attempting to adjust to erratic production of hormones by the ovaries.

When a woman's menstrual periods have stopped occurring altogether she has reached menopause and her ovaries have almost entirely stopped producing hormones. Other physical changes may also begin to take place.

WHAT PHYSICAL CHANGES MIGHT A WOMAN EXPERIENCE ONCE HER PERIODS HAVE STOPPED?

The intermediate signs of menopause may include:

- Vaginal dryness that can result in painful intercourse and lead to a loss of sexual interest.

- Urinary changes may lead to increased frequency and urgency to urinate or to urinary tract infections.

- Vaginal and bladder infections may occur more frequently.

- Lower abdominal congestion can cause bloating, difficult digestion, constipation, and hemorrhoids. These conditions may be accompanied by headaches.

- Mucous membranes of the vagina and vulva may become fragile and prone to being easily damaged or may bleed during intercourse.

- Appearance changes may become obvious, including body shape changes, skin that is dryer and begins to wrinkle, and fingernails that break more easily.

- Breasts may change, begin to lose their buoyancy, and start to droop. They may become sore or develop hypersensitive masses. Because the onset of breast disease is common at this time, mammograms are recommended by the American Cancer Society.

WHAT CAUSES THESE INTERMEDIATE SIGNS OF MENOPAUSE?

Now that the ovaries are no longer producing hormones, cells, tissues, and organs within the body that were supported and stimulated by those hormones are adjusting to the change.

During this time a woman's dietary and lifestyle habits can enhance her future health and reduce the chances of her developing more serious health problems that occur after menopause.

WHAT ARE THE LONG-TERM EFFECTS OF MENOPAUSE ON A WOMAN'S BODY?

Postmenopausal physical changes may include:

- Pelvic organ atrophy leading to sagging internal tissues and organs, including the uterus, vagina, and bladder.

- Bone changes, depending on the condition of a woman's bones and connective tissue and her capacity to retain and absorb calcium, could include aches and pains in joints, fallen arches of the feet, or pinched disks between the spinal vertebrae. Extreme bone changes can lead to osteoporosis.

- Circulatory changes that may be evident in varicose veins or feelings of heaviness and cramping in the legs. Extreme circulatory changes could lead to high blood pressure, heart disease, or stroke.

DOES EVERY WOMAN EXPERIENCE ALL OF THESE SIGNS OF MENOPAUSE?

Every woman with an intact uterus will eventually stop having menstrual periods and most women experience a change in their menstrual periods before they stop entirely. The most common complaints of women during menopause are hot flashes and vaginal dryness, although some women pass through menopause without experiencing any discomfort.

The likelihood of a woman's experiencing later signs of menopause, which may lead to serious health disorders and disease, is based on each woman's personal health status, her family history, and her lifestyle and dietary habits during menopause and into later life.

AT WHAT AGE DOES MENOPAUSE BEGIN?

Menopause usually begins between the ages of 48 and 52. Obvious hormonal changes such as irritability, mood swings, sleep disturbances, changes in memory retention, and aches and pains, can begin as early as 35 or 40—five to ten years before the actual onset of menopause. This is especially true for women who suffer from PMS, ovarian cysts, endometriosis, fibroid tumors, or other disorders associated with female hormone imbalances.

An early menopause may occur during a woman's early forties. Premature menopause (loss of ovarian hormone production before the age of 40) has been known to occur, although rarely, in women as young as 20.

WHAT CAUSES PREMATURE MENOPAUSE?

Surgical removal of the ovaries certainly causes premature menopause, but a woman with intact ovaries may also experience premature menopause for various reasons. Some are born with fewer eggs than normal, so their ovaries stop producing estrogen earlier than the average.

Other women may experience premature menopause from surgery that cuts off the supply of blood to the ovaries, from chemotherapy or radiation treatments for cancer, or because severe infections have damaged the ovaries or destroyed ovarian tissue.

HOW LONG DOES THE MENOPAUSAL TRANSITION LAST?

The average period of time during which a woman is aware of her menopausal transition is usually five to seven years, although some women may not know for sure when it starts or when it's over.

AT WHAT AGE DOES MENOPAUSE USUALLY OCCUR?

Every woman is different. The average age that natural menopause occurs is around age 50 or 51, but it may occur as early as age 35 or as late as age 55.

Women who have not gone through menopause naturally and have their ovaries surgically removed go through menopause immediately.

WHY DOES EVERY WOMAN GO THROUGH NATURAL MENOPAUSE AT A DIFFERENT AGE?

Many factors influence the age at which menopause begins in each woman, as well as affecting her degree of discomfort and the eventual development of menopause-related health problems. Among them: heredity, hormone production, overall health, lifestyle factors including diet, exercise, stress, alcohol intake, smoking and toxin exposure, and the altitude at which she lives.

HOW DO GENES INFLUENCE WHEN A WOMAN WILL GO THROUGH MENOPAUSE?

It is obvious by looking at our biological families that we have similar genetic material revealed by our body type, skin color, hair color, and more. Often our genetic makeup also indicates a pattern of hormonal function within our body as well, which may translate to menopausal pattern similarities among our female biological forebears, our female siblings, and ourselves. However, menopausal patterns may also be influenced by lifestyle patterns passed from generation to generation, such as diet, stress management, physical activity, smoking, drinking, and environmental toxin exposure.

DOES THAT MEAN A WOMAN WILL GO THROUGH MENOPAUSE AT ABOUT THE SAME AGE AS HER MOTHER, GRANDMOTHERS, AND OLDER SISTERS?

Because the quality of life has changed dramatically during the last century, with life expectancy increasing, a woman today may not go through menopause at exactly the same age as her mother and grandmothers. But even considering other factors, a genetic predisposition toward early or late menopause may show up.

HOW DOES A WOMAN'S OVERALL HEALTH INFLUENCE THE AGE AND CONDITIONS OF HER MENOPAUSE?

Ovaries are glands that interact with various other glands, which make up the endocrine system located throughout the body. Secretions from these glands stimulate and support every part of your body. When one of these glands stops producing hormones, it affects all the rest. The body then attempts to rebalance itself naturally. If a woman's body does not need to expend energy overcoming existing health problems then it can adjust more easily to the changes of menopause.

HOW DO DIET AND EXERCISE AFFECT MENOPAUSE?

A healthy diet and regular exercise can enhance a woman's overall health, especially during and after menopause. Positive changes in nutritional intake, exercise, and other lifestyle factors can have a surprisingly beneficial effect on the way a woman feels during menopause and on into later life. See chapter 6 for information about lifestyle changes that can help make the menopausal transition easier with or without *HRT.*

HOW DOES STRESS AFFECT MENOPAUSE?

Negative stress can be detrimental to a woman's health at any time of her life. But unmanaged stress during menopause can increase a woman's hormone imbalances, enhancing emotional and physical discomforts she may already be feeling. Unchecked, this pattern can have a destructive effect on her future health, especially her skeletal and cardiovascular systems. Chapter 6 offers suggestions for how you can reduce the impact of negative stress on your health.

HOW DOES ALCOHOL CONSUMPTION AFFECT MENOPAUSE?

Women who regularly consume substantial amounts of alcoholic beverages go through menopause earlier than those who do not. Excessive alcohol consumption is detrimental to any woman's overall health.

WHY DOES SMOKING INFLUENCE MENOPAUSE?

Besides the other damage cigarette smoking does to a woman's body, studies suggest that smoking also affects her estrogen levels. Reports indicate that smokers go through menopause one to two years earlier than nonsmokers or exsmokers. The longer a woman has smoked and the number of cigarettes she smoked daily seems to move her closer to an early menopause. Women who live with smokers and are exposed to passive cigarette smoke also seem to enter menopause earlier, as do women whose mothers smoked.

Smokers are also at higher risk for developing health problems during their postmenopausal years, including osteoporosis and cardiovascular diseases and disorders.

HOW DOES TOXIC EXPOSURE AFFECT MENOPAUSE?

We are only beginning to understand how exposure to toxic substances affects a woman's health, but the news is not good. Contact with chemicals in soil and water are being linked to higher risks of developing breast cancer, endometriosis, and osteoporosis, as well as being generally detrimental to a woman's overall health.

WHAT DOES THE ALTITUDE AT WHICH A WOMAN LIVES HAVE TO DO WITH HER MENOPAUSE?

Although the reasons are not clear, studies have shown that women who live at high altitudes enter menopausal transition years earlier than women who live at lower altitudes.

DOES MENOPAUSE CAUSE SERIOUS HEALTH PROBLEMS?

Menopause is a natural physical transition and does not necessarily cause serious health problems, although problems generally do develop during the middle and later years of life. Because menopause has a dramatic effect within a woman's body, women who are healthier during menopause usually have fewer health problems afterward.

DOES MENOPAUSE REQUIRE MEDICAL TREATMENT?

At least 50 percent of women do nothing about menopause because they consider it a normal transition in life.

Women most likely to seek medical assistance during

menopause are those experiencing severe menopausal discomfort or those at risk for developing serious health conditions that can occur during the middle and later years of life when hormone production changes.

DOES MENOPAUSE HAVE LONG-TERM EFFECTS ON YOUR HEALTH?

Diminished hormone production may lead to pelvic organ atrophy, osteoporosis, and increased risk of heart attack. However, these long-term effects can be offset by dietary adjustments, lifestyle changes, and hormone replacement therapy when it's appropriate.

▲ ▲ ▲

CHAPTER 2

What Is Hormone Replacement Therapy (HRT)?

Hormone replacement is not as simple as taking a pill once a day for the rest of your life. There are various ways for supplying hormones to your body during and after menopause, as well as numerous types of hormones available. Only when a woman has as much information and medical advice as possible can she decide which type of *HRT* could work best for her.

WHAT IS HORMONE REPLACEMENT THERAPY (HRT)*?*

HRT is a physician-prescribed program of treatment for women who are experiencing hormonal imbalances, usually during and after menopause. *HRT* may consist of estrogen alone (ERT) or estrogen, progestins, natural progesterone, or testosterone in various combinations (all considered *HRT*).

WHY IS HRT *PRESCRIBED BY DOCTORS?*

HRT has been shown to alleviate the hot flashes, mood swings, and vaginal dryness some women experience during menopause. *HRT* also appears to reduce the risks of osteoporosis, heart disease, and pelvic organ atrophy during and after menopause by regulating a woman's hormone production.

WHEN WAS HRT *FIRST INTRODUCED?*

Estrogen replacement therapy was introduced to the American public in the early 1960s as a treatment for discomfort associated with menopause. By the mid 1970s, millions of women were taking estrogen.

ESTROGEN

WHAT IS ESTROGEN?

Estrogen, which acts as a cellular stimulant, is a hormone manufactured naturally by a woman's body. Three types of estrogen are produced by your body: your ovaries produce estradiol, the strongest estrogen, which contributes to monthly ovulation and normal menstrual cycles; a less potent estrogen, estrone, is converted from elements of fatty tissue; and an even weaker estrogen, estriol, results from estradiol and estrone metabolism within your body.

Synthetic estrogen was first isolated in laboratory studies during the 1920s.

WHERE DOES THE ESTROGEN WOMEN TAKE COME FROM?

The estrogens prescribed for women can either be naturally derived or synthetically produced. Estrone and estradiol are the two types of estrogen used most often. Less potent forms of natural estrogen, called phytoestrogens, are derived from estrogens in plants. Estriol is a phytoestrogen used for HRT.

The brand name *Premarin* is one of the most popular forms of estrogen prescribed for menopausal and postmenopausal women, and is, in fact, the most prescribed medication in the United States. It is considered a natural estrogen because it is manufactured from the urine of pregnant mares. However, many alternative health care professionals say although it is natural to horses, it is not natural to women.

There is further controversy surrounding *Premarin* because of the way it is produced. Female horses raised on "estrogen farms" are kept continually pregnant and confined. After giving birth, male foals are destroyed because they cannot support the production of urine used to make *Premarin*. Animal rights activists are fighting to enact programs to resolve these conditions which they consider cruelty. While they have not been successful in changing the conditions under which pregnant mares are housed, they have successfully created male foal adoption programs.

DO NATURAL ESTROGENS AND SYNTHETIC ESTROGENS HAVE DIFFERENT EFFECTS IN THE BODY?

Natural estrogens are not as potent as most synthetic estrogens and appear to cause fewer side effects in women. The more potent synthetic estrogens suppress ovulation and are usually prescribed in birth control pills, not for menopausal and postmenopausal use.

The biggest concern about taking estrogen is the increased risk of cancer, which is associated with estrone and estradiol. However, *estriol*, the weakest form of estrogen, does *not* increase the risk of cancer and is even believed to protect the body against cancer.

IS ESTROGEN ALWAYS TAKEN IN PILL FORM?

Estrogen can be taken in various ways: orally in pill form, by injection into muscles or veins, inserted vaginally with suppositories or creams, or absorbed through the skin from patches.

IS IT BETTER TO TAKE ESTROGEN ORALLY?

Taking estrogen orally is the most common choice of women, probably because it is most often prescribed by doctors and it is easy and convenient. But this form can have both positive and negative effects.

For oral estrogen to be most effective it must be adequately absorbed by the intestines and pass through the liver to enter a woman's general circulation. However, some women may not adequately absorb estrogen through the intestines and will need to take higher doses for the estrogen to be effective. Taking more potent doses of oral estrogen may increase their side effects.

17

WHAT ARE THE NEGATIVE EFFECTS
OF TAKING ESTROGEN ORALLY?

Because oral estrogen passes through the liver, it stimulates the production of proteins that may increase blood pressure, interfere with blood clotting, or negatively affect the gallbladder. Although uncommon, these are documented side effects when oral doses of estrogen are too high for the body to utilize positively.

Estrogen replacement drugs may lower zinc levels and increase copper levels in the blood. Zinc deficiencies can lead to depression, copper elevation can increase moodiness.

WHAT ESTROGEN PILLS ARE
GENERALLY PRESCRIBED?

Oral forms of natural estrogens produced outside the human body and prescribed for *HRT* include conjugated equine estrogen (*Premarin*), estrone sulfate (*Ogen*), esterified estrogens (*Estratab*), estradiol valerate (*Progynova*), and micronized estradiol (*Estrace*).

The synthetic oral estrogens most commonly used in birth control pills are ethinyl estradiol (*Estinyl*), quinestrol (*Estrovis*), and diethylstilbestrol (*DES*).

WHY WOULD A WOMAN CHOOSE
ESTROGEN INJECTIONS?

Estrogen injections are sometimes used when a woman cannot tolerate oral estrogen intake to prevent hot flashes and other negative effects of menopause while recovering from surgery that included removal of the ovaries. Estrogen injections have the advantage of being absorbed directly into the body's circulation without passing through the stomach, intestines, and liver.

However, there are numerous disadvantages to estrogen injections, the most obvious being the discomfort and inconvenience of the shots. After injection there can be an initial high level of estrogen metabolism by the body, followed by an uncontrollable diminishing supply. If a woman experiences the side effects sometimes associated with estrogen intake (discussed in chapter 3), there is no way to counteract them and it may take three or four weeks before they subside. Other forms of estrogen offer a woman better control and quicker withdrawal if she desires it.

Since its development, the estrogen skin patch, *Estraderm*, is usually used when injections were in the past.

WHEN ELSE WOULD THE ESTROGEN SKIN PATCH BE PREFERRED?

The *Estraderm* skin patch provides a natural form of estrogen, (17-B estradiol) that enables a woman's body to absorb estrogen without its passing through the stomach, intestines, and liver. Therefore, the risks associated with liver disease, gallbladder disease, high blood pressure, and blood clotting are decreased. Consequently, transdermal application of *HRT* is becoming more popular, although it is not as easy or convenient as taking pills.

The estrogen skin patch is applied twice a week and slowly releases estrogen into the body just as the ovaries would if they were present or functioning. The patch has been shown to alleviate the discomforts of menopause such as hot flashes and may be considered for postmenopausal osteoporosis prevention.

WHY WOULD A WOMAN NOT CHOOSE THE ESTROGEN SKIN PATCH?

Estrogen applied to the skin does not offer the heart disease protective benefits of oral estrogens because estrogen must pass through the liver for that organ to release proteins that raise beneficial HDL-cholesterol levels in the blood. Some women experience skin irritation from wearing the patch. Further, the skin patch only provides estrogen to the body and will not benefit women who select a combination estrogen/progesterone therapy unless natural progesterone is used at the same time.

WHEN WOULD A WOMAN CHOOSE
VAGINAL APPLICATION OF ESTROGEN?

The absorption of estrogen vaginally is usually not reliable enough to be considered for estrogen replacement therapy. However, vaginal applications of estrogen can be helpful for women who choose not to take estrogen replacement therapy but still desire the benefits estrogen can offer for vaginal dryness and atrophy.

HOW OFTEN CAN ESTROGEN BE APPLIED VAGINALLY?

The needs of every woman differ. For some, a small amount of estrogen cream inserted into the vagina once a week may be enough to relieve dryness; others may require application three times a week.

Estrogen cream can be used vaginally along with other types of *HRT*, but since vaginally applied estrogen is also absorbed into the system to some degree, you should discuss your personal treatment program with your physician.

WHAT VAGINAL ESTROGEN
CREAMS ARE MOST COMMONLY USED?

The estrogen creams available for vaginal application include: conjugated equine estrogen (*Premarin*), estropipate (*Ogen*), dinestrol (DV cream estragard), and estradiol cream (*Estrace*), and diethylstibestrol (generic).

HOW DOES A WOMAN KNOW IF SHE IS TAKING
THE RIGHT AMOUNT OF ESTROGEN?

Adequate levels of estrogen intake are indicated by relief of menopausal and postmenopausal discomforts such as hot flashes, night sweats, and vaginal dryness.

Using estrogen in any form requires regular, periodic monitoring by your physician, as discussed in chapter 4.

If you are uncertain about the effectiveness of your choice of estrogen intake, your doctor may suggest the following laboratory tests:

- Your vaginal estrogen levels can be determined by analyzing a vaginal smear.

- Your blood cholesterol levels can be monitored to assess heart disease risk status.

- Your estrogen blood levels can be monitored to determine if you are absorbing enough estrogen into your circulation.

- Your osteoporosis status and bone loss can be evaluated with periodic bone density measurements.

NATURAL PROGESTERONE AND PROGESTINS

WHAT IS PROGESTERONE?

Progesterone is a hormone manufactured by your ovaries. It is an intermediate building block for other hormones within the female body. During premenopausal years the cyclic increase and decrease in progesterone triggers the endometrial shedding known as a menstrual period. When your body produces abnormal levels of progesterone your menstrual cycles will become irregular.

WHERE DOES THE PROGESTERONE WOMEN TAKE COME FROM?

Progesterone was first isolated in 1934. During the 1950s it was discovered that at least 1,000 plants contain progesterone substances. Three types of progesterone are used in hormone replacement therapy:

- progestins, also called progestogens, progestational agents, or gestagens, are produced synthetically from natural progesterone. They include medroxyprogesterone acetate (*Provera, Amen, Cycrin, Curretabs*), megesterol acetate (*Megace*), and 17-a hydroxyprogesterone caproate (*Delalutin*).

- progestins manufactured from testosterone include dimethisterone, ethynodiol diacetate, orethindrone (*Micronor, Nor-Q.D., Norlutin*), norethindrone acetate, northynodrel (*Aygestin, Norlutate*), norgestrel (*Ovrette*), and 1-norgestrel.

21

- natural progesterone (diosgenin) is usually derived from Mexican yams (dioscorea). *Pro-Gest* is the product most commonly used.

WHY ARE PROGESTINS USED IN HRT ALONG WITH ESTROGEN?

In the beginning, estrogen alone was the recommended treatment for most menopausal and postmenopausal women. But by the mid 1970s studies began to indicate that women taking estrogen alone were five times more likely to develop uterine cancer and breast cancer. Subsequent studies showed that taking progestins along with the estrogen for at least ten days each month reduced the incidence of uterine cancer.

The use of progesterone in hormone replacement therapy can restore the natural estrogen/progesterone balance in a woman's body. Because progesterone has a beneficial effect on the uterus, adding progesterone to *HRT* reduces the risk of endometrial and uterine cancer caused by excessive estrogen. Therefore, women who still have a uterus during and after menopause are advised to add progestins or natural progesterone to their treatment program when choosing hormone replacement therapy.

HOW ARE PROGESTINS TAKEN?

Progestins can be taken in the same ways as estrogens: orally, vaginally, rectally, and by injection.

IF YOUR UTERUS HAS BEEN REMOVED, DO YOU NEED TO TAKE PROGESTINS?

If a woman's uterus has been removed (hysterectomy), progestins are generally not recommended because they have been shown to have negative side effects.

WHAT SIDE EFFECTS CAN OCCUR WHEN A WOMAN TAKES PROGESTINS?

Some progestins appear to have the opposite effect of estrogen on the HDL-cholesterol levels of the body, causing beneficial cholesterol to be lowered, possibly offsetting the benefits of estrogen against heart disease risk.

Progestins taken with estrogen cyclically simulate the natural rise and fall of hormones in the premenopausal menstrual cycle and may cause a return of monthly menstrual bleeding. This side effect can be eliminated with lower doses of progestins or by taking progestins every two or three months, rather than monthly on a cyclical schedule.

Some studies indicate progestins may increase a woman's risks for breast cancer. Although not as common, other possible side effects of progestins may include anxiety, depression, moodiness, nervousness, headaches, and abdominal bloating.

CAN PROGESTINS WITHOUT ESTROGEN RELIEVE MENOPAUSAL DISCOMFORT?

Progestins have been shown to relieve hot flashes for women who cannot take estrogen because they have medical conditions that would be exacerbated by estrogen intake.

However, women taking progestins alone cannot count on improvement of vaginal dryness or protection against heart disease.

WHEN WOULD PROGESTINS WITHOUT ESTROGEN BE TAKEN?

Women with breast or endometrial cancer are usually advised to avoid estrogen therapy, as are women with breast fibroids or uterine fibroids because these estrogen-dependent conditions may worsen when estrogen is taken.

WHAT'S THE DIFFERENCE IN THE PROGESTINS PRESCRIBED IN HRT?

The medroxyprogesterone acetate progestins (*Amen, Curretabs, Cycrin, and Provera*) are often favored by physicians prescribing *HRT* because they seem to have the least detrimental effect on blood cholesterol levels.

When progestins were first added to estrogen in *HRT*, they were derived from the hormones testosterone and 19-nortestosterone. Although they are still prescribed, these progestational agents may have an androgenic effect in women, resulting in masculine-like symptoms such as weight gain and muscle development, oily skin and acne, unwanted hair growth, lowering of the voice, and enlargement of the clitoris. Stronger doses may also have a more negative effect on blood cholesterol levels, increasing the risk of heart disease.

WHEN ARE THE PROGESTINS DERIVED FROM TESTOSTERONE USED?

Progestins derived from testosterone are often used in birth control pills along with estrogen. The progesterone-only birth control pills (*Micronor* and *Ovrette*) prescribed for women who cannot take estrogen contain testosterone derivatives, as does levonorgestrel, the hormone used in *Norplant*, the contraceptive implant.

The testosterone-derived progestin, norethindrone, is being used for postmenopausal treatment because the lower dosage has been shown to cause fewer side effects.

WHAT'S THE DIFFERENCE BETWEEN NATURAL PROGESTERONE AND PROGESTINS?

Natural progesterone is identical in molecular structure to the progesterone manufactured by the body. Progestins are synthetically produced by modifying the molecular structure of progesterone derived from plants or from testosterone. Once the progesterone molecule is synthetically altered in a laboratory, it becomes a progestin and is no longer considered natural progesterone. Therefore, the distinction between natural progesterone and progestins is important when discussing and considering hormone replacement therapy.

DO NATURAL PROGESTERONE AND PROGESTINS ACT DIFFERENTLY IN THE BODY?

Because natural progesterone is identical in molecular structure to progesterone produced by the body, it performs the same role within the body's complicated hormonal interaction. Progestins do not all have the same effects in the body.

For the purposes of hormone replacement therapy, both have the same beneficial effect on the endometrium, protecting the uterine lining and possibly triggering menstrual flow. However, progestins have been shown to have side effects within the body and it has been reported that natural progesterone does not appear to have any significant side effects. For these reasons, the use of natural progesterone in hormone replacement therapy has recently become more popular.

HOW IS NATURAL PROGESTERONE TAKEN?

Natural progesterone can be taken orally, supplied to the body transdermally by massaging a cream containing diosgenin into the skin, or sublingually by holding under the tongue a vitamin E oil-based diosgenin.

IS NATURAL PROGESTERONE USED ALONE OR WITH ESTROGEN?

Natural progesterone is commonly used alone in the treatment of PMS before menopause. It can be used alone during perimenopause when a woman's body may have excessive estrogen effects, causing uterine or breast problems. After menopause it is usually used with an estrogen.

HOW IS NATURAL PROGESTERONE BENEFICIAL FOR A WOMAN'S BODY?

Advocates of natural progesterone have found it very effective in relieving both PMS and the discomfort of menopause. It is also claimed to reduce the risk of other serious health conditions that women develop after menopause such as heart disease and osteoporosis, and has been shown to stimulate formation of new bone in women with osteoporosis.

DOES NATURAL PROGESTERONE HAVE ANY SIDE EFFECTS?

Just as with progestins, a woman's menstrual period may return or periodic spotting or breakthrough bleeding may occur. Natural progesterone may also increase thyroid activity somewhat, a possible concern for women who take thyroid medication.

WHY ARE PROGESTINS MORE WIDELY USED IN HRT THAN NATURAL PROGESTERONE?

Progestin/estrogen combinations are packaged by large drug companies, making progestins taken orally easier and more convenient.

Natural progesterone in *HRT* is a fairly recent development. Most doctors are more familiar with progestins because they learn about them in medical school and because the large drug companies promote the use of their products that contain progestins. However, the benefits of natural progesterone are beginning to be more widely recognized by physicians.

At this time, medical documentation of the use of natural progesterone is considered anecdotal, because it is being used without double blind studies for comparison. Scientifically designed studies usually result for two reasons: Before a drug can be approved by the FDA (Food and Drug Administration) for general use it must undergo extensive scientific medical study. After

FDA approval, many drug companies underwrite usage studies in order to promote the sale of their products.

Because the molecular structure of natural progesterone is not altered, it is considered a natural substance, not a drug. It cannot be patented by drug companies and no prescription is required for its purchase. As a result, extensive drug testing has not been done using natural progesterone for the purpose of FDA approval and there is no benefit for drug companies to underwrite studies to promote a product they cannot patent and which can be easily produced.

IS THERE A NATURAL ESTROGEN/PROGESTERONE COMBINATION AVAILABLE ON THE MARKET?

Your doctor can prescribe an estrogen/natural progesterone combination derived from plant sources. The oral form contains natural progesterone with tri-estrogen, which is 80 percent estriol (phytoestrogen), 10 percent estrone, and 10 percent estradiol. A phytoestrogen/natural progesterone cream (*Ostaderm*) and gel are also available for topical or vaginal application.

HOW IS A PHYTOESTROGEN/NATURAL PROGESTERONE CREAM OR GEL USED?

A phytoestrogen/natural progesterone cream or gel is applied to skin, usually on the stomach, until menopausal discomfort stops. It can be used the entire month, if necessary, except the last four or five days. It can also be inserted vaginally.

ARE THERE SIDE EFFECTS FROM USING PHYTOESTROGEN/NATURAL PROGESTERONE CREAMS OR GELS?

A woman's menstrual period may continue or return, just as it may when she takes any *HRT* that includes natural progesterone or a progestin in any form.

WHY WOULD A WOMAN USE A PHYTOESTROGEN/NATURAL PROGESTERONE COMBINATION INSTEAD OF OTHER TYPES OF HRT?

Some women prefer a more natural and gentle approach to their health care.

The tri-estrogen/natural progesterone combination has been shown to be effective in relieving a woman's menopausal discomforts while it eliminates her risks of cancer and protects her bone health.

A woman who has taken *Premarin* and/or *Provera* and has experienced side effects may elect to switch to the phytoestrogen/natural progesterone combination.

WHY DON'T MORE DOCTORS SUGGEST WOMEN USE THE PHYTOESTROGEN/NATURAL PROGESTERONE COMBINATION?

For reasons similar to those for doctors not suggesting the use of natural progesterone. Because the tri-estrogen/natural progesterone combination is not manufactured by a large drug company that promotes its products, it is not as widely available or as well known within the conventional medical community. Doctors who seek to offer alternative or combination conventional/alternative treatment programs are more likely to be familiar with the natural hormones, their uses, and benefits. The Suggested Reading List and Resources appendix provide sources for information on the natural hormones that you may choose to share with your doctor.

TESTOSTERONE

WHAT IS TESTOSTERONE?

Testosterone is generally considered a male hormone because it is abundantly produced by the bodies of men. However, a small quantity of testosterone is also produced by the ovaries of women. Interestingly, the testosterone in both women and men is converted to estrogen in the brain before being used by the body.

WHY WOULD A WOMAN CHOOSE TO TAKE TESTOSTERONE FOR MENOPAUSE?

The small amount of testosterone released by the ovaries prior to menopause appears to influence the energy level and sex drive of women. When testosterone is added to estrogen in *HRT* it seems to serve that same function in menopausal and postmenopausal women, adding to a feeling of well being.

IS TESTOSTERONE USED IN HRT INSTEAD OF PROGESTINS?

Because testosterone does not protect the uterine lining, as natural progesterone or progestins will do, it is not prescribed as *HRT* instead of progestins for a woman whose uterus is intact. A woman who has had a hysterectomy may be advised to take a testosterone-estrogen combination during and after menopause.

WHAT TESTOSTERONE-ESTROGEN COMBINATIONS ARE USUALLY PRESCRIBED DURING AND AFTER MENOPAUSE?

Estratest and *Premarin* with methyltestosterone can be taken orally. *Premarin*, the stronger of the two, is more likely to cause side effects in women. The lower dosage Estratest has been shown to be more beneficial overall.

The testosterone-estrogen combination is also available by injection (*Depo-testadiol*).

TAKING HORMONES

HOW OFTEN IS HRT TAKEN?

HRT may be taken in a cycle or continuously.

In cyclic therapy estrogen is taken most of the month with a progestin or natural progesterone added for 10 to 13 days only, to duplicate the natural hormonal cycles of healthy premenopausal women.

In continuous therapy both estrogen and a progestin are taken together the same number of days each month.

HOW IS CYCLIC HRT TAKEN?

There are two ways to take *HRT* in a cycle: Estrogen alone is taken during the first 12 days of the month, then beginning the 13th day progestin or natural progesterone is taken along with estrogen through the 25th day of the month. Finally, no medication is taken for the rest of the month, which duplicates a woman's normal menstrual cycle.

However, some women experience headaches and hot flashes during the five or six days they do not take the estrogen. If that happens, a woman may choose to take estrogen every day of the month with a progestin or natural progesterone added for 10 to 13 days each month, usually the first 10 to 13 days.

For a woman who can take estrogen and who chooses to do so, it is important to add a progestin or natural progesterone for a period of time during the month to protect the uterine lining if her uterus is intact.

WHAT ARE THE DISADVANTAGES OF CYCLIC HRT?

Many women continue to have a monthly period even after menopause. To eliminate this side effect of cyclic *HRT* some women may prefer continuous *HRT*.

WILL A WOMAN'S MENSTRUAL PERIOD CONTINUE AS LONG AS SHE TAKES HRT CYCLICALLY?

Most women with an intact uterus taking cyclic *HRT* still have a menstrual period even after menopause because the sudden drop in the progestin or natural progesterone causes shedding of the uterine lining. However, their periods will probably be lighter than before and will gradually decrease over time.

The effects of *HRT* on your pelvic organs and the significance of abnormal bleeding are discussed in chapter 12.

HOW IS CONTINUOUS HRT TAKEN?

Continuous *HRT* can be taken in two ways. A women takes estrogen plus a very low dosage of a progestin every day of the month or she takes the estrogen-progestin combination five days a week, with weekends off.

WHY WOULD A WOMAN CHOOSE CONTINUOUS HRT?

Continuous *HRT* can eliminate the menstrual bleeding many women find undesirable after menopause. It protects the uterine lining with lower doses of progestins than those usually required in cyclic therapy.

WHAT ARE THE DISADVANTAGES OF CONTINUOUS HRT?

Sometimes breakthrough bleeding still occurs, requiring adjustment in the progestin dosage until the right balance is achieved.

Although lower levels of progestins may be taken during continuous *HRT*, progestins may still have a negative effect on blood cholesterol levels and increase the risk of heart disease, as discussed in chapter 11.

IS CONTINUOUS HRT BETTER FOR SOME WOMEN THAN OTHERS?

Until the completion of menopause a woman's ovaries are still producing hormones to some degree, often irregularly, making it difficult to regulate *HRT* intake. Therefore, women who have completed menopause generally find continuous *HRT* more comfortable and beneficial.

IF A WOMAN IS TAKING PROGESTINS WITH ESTROGEN, CAN SHE SWITCH TO NATURAL PROGESTERONE WITH ESTROGEN INSTEAD?

If you are taking progestins with estrogen and want to switch, you need to tell your doctor. Some doctors may still not be aware of the benefits of natural progesterone and phytoestrogen, so you may need to suggest sources of information such as those in the Suggested Reading List and Resources appendix.

IF A WOMAN IS TAKING HRT AND WANTS TO DISCONTINUE, CAN SHE JUST STOP TAKING IT ONE DAY?

If you are taking *HRT* and want to stop, it is best to inform your doctor of your decision so a program can be devised for gradual withdrawal by prescribing lower and lower doses of hormones or by scheduling you to skip days during the months you continue with *HRT*.

If you are using a skin patch, you can wear it for gradually shorter periods of time and less often.

WHAT ARE THE NAMES AND DOSAGES OF THE VARIOUS HORMONES ON THE MARKET?

ESTROGENS

Estrogens taken orally (pill form):

Estinyl (ethinyl estradiol), manufactured by Schering in dosages of .02 mg, .05 mg, and .5 mg.

Estrace (micronized estradiol), manufactured by Mead Johnson in dosages of 1.0 mg and 2.0 mg.

Estratab (esterified estrogens), manufactured by Solvay in dosages of 0.3 mg, 0.625 mg, 1.25 mg, and 2.5 mg.

Estrovis (quinestrol), manufactured by Parke-Davis in a dosage of 0.1 mg.

Ogen (estropipate), manufactured by Abbott in dosages of 0.625 mg, 1.25 mg, 2.5 mg, and 5.0 mg.

Premarin (conjugated estrogens), manufactured by Wyeth-Ayerst in dosages of 0.3 mg, 0.625 mg, 0.9 mg, 1.25 mg, and 2.5 mg.

Tace (chlorotrianisene), manufactured by Merrill-Dow in dosages of 12 mg, 25 mg, and 72 mg.

Estrogens available for muscular injection:

Delestrogen (estradiol valerate), manufactured by Squibb in dosages of 10 mg/ml, 20 mg/ml, and 40 mg/ml.

Depo-Estradiol (estradiol cypionate), manufactured by Upjohn in dosages of 1 mg/ml and 5 mg/ml.

Estraval (estradiol valerate), manufactured by Solvay in dosages of 10 mg/ml and 20 mg/ml.

Estrogen for muscular or intravenous injection:

Premarin (conjugated estrogens), manufactured by Wyeth-Ayerst in a 25 mg vial dosage.

Estrogen in a skin patch:

Estraderm (transdermal), manufactured by Ciba-Geigy in a dosage of 0.05 mg.

Estrogen vaginal creams:

Estrace vaginal cream (17-beta-estradiol), manufactured by Mead Johnson.

Estragard cream (dienestrol), manufactured by Solvay.

Ogen vaginal cream (estropipate), manufactured by Abbott.

Ortho dienestrol cream (dienestrol), manufactured by Ortho.

Premarin vaginal cream (conjugated estrogens), manufactured by Wyeth-Ayerst.

Estrogen in suppository:

Diethylstilbestrol suppositories (diethylstilbestrol), manufactured by Lilly.

PROGESTINS

Progestins taken orally (pill form):

Amen (medroxyprogesterone acetate), manufactured by Carnick in a dosage of 10 mg.

Aygestin (norethindrone acetate), manufactured by Wyeth-Ayerst in a dosage of 5 mg.

Curretabs (medroxyprogesterone acetate), manufactured by

Solvay in a dosage of 10 mg.

Cycrin (medroxyprogesterone acetate), manufactured by Wyeth-Ayerst in a dosage of 10 mg.

Megace (megesterol acetate), manufactured by Bristol-Myers in dosages of 20 mg and 40 mg.

Micronor (norethindrone), manufactured by Ortho in a dosage of 0.35 mg.

Norlutate (norethindrone acetate), manufactured by Parke-Davis in a dosage of 5 mg.

Norlutin (norethindrone), manufactured by Parke-Davis in a dosage of 5 mg.

Nor-Q.D. (norethindrone), manufactured by Syntex in a dosage of 0.35 mg.

Ovrette (norgestrel), manufactured by Wyeth-Ayerst in a dosage of 0.075 mg.

Provera (medroxyprogesterone acetate), manufactured by Upjohn in dosages of 2.5 mg, 5 mg, and 10 mg.

ESTROGEN + TESTOSTERONE COMBINATIONS

Estrogen + testosterone combination taken orally (pill form):

Estratest (esterified estrogens), manufactured by Solvay in dosages of 1.25 mg + 2.5 mg, 0.625 mg + 1.25 mg.

Premarin with methyl testosterone (conjugated estrogens + methyl testosterone), manufactured by Wyeth-Ayerst in dosages of 0.625 mg + 5.0 mg, 1.25 mg + 10 mg.

Estrogen + testosterone combination for injection:

Depo-Testadiol injectable (estradiol cypionate + testosterone cypionate), manufactured by Upjohn in a dosage of 2 mg + 50 mg.

PHYTOESTROGEN/NATURAL PROGESTERONE COMBINATION

Tri-estrogen (80% phytoestrogen estriol, 10% estrace, 10% estradiol) with natural progesterone capsules, cream, or gel are formulated by the Women's International Pharmacy to suit a woman's individual needs as prescribed by her doctor (see appendix).

Ostaderm cream for transdermal application, manufactured by Bezwecken Transdermals, contains both plant-derived estrogens and progesterone.

NATURAL PROGESTERONE

Natural progesterone cream for transdermal or vaginal use:

Pro-Gest, manufactured by Professional and Technical Services, diosgenin derived from wild Mexican yam (dioscorea) roots.

Natural orogesterone oil for sublingual or vaginal use:

Pro-Gest, manufactured by Professional and Technical Services, diosgenin extract of wild Mexican yam (dioscorea) roots.

Because new products are periodically introduced to the market, this list may not include newer supplemental hormones introduced by pharmaceutical companies or those developed by manufacturers of natural hormones.

CHAPTER 3

What Are The Positive and Negative Aspects of Hormone Replacement Therapy?

It is important for every woman to understand the positive and negative effects that different types of hormones used as *HRT* might have on her body. This information will enable you to assess realistically your own personal needs, desires, and expected results when you consider whether *HRT* is right for you and to assist you in deciding which type of hormones to take.

WHAT ARE THE BENEFITS OF ESTROGEN REPLACEMENT FOR MENOPAUSAL AND POSTMENOPAUSAL WOMEN?

Estrogen usually relieves the discomforts associated with menopause, such as hot flashes and any accompanying night sweats, heart palpitations, and sleep disturbances, as well as vaginal dryness. It is also believed to reduce a woman's rate of skin wrinkling. These benefits often result in an increased feeling of well-being, vitality, and sexuality, thus alleviating the anxiety, nervousness, mood changes, and depression some women experience during menopause.

Estrogen replacement has also been shown to influence these more serious health problems in women:

- It can reduce the risk of osteoporosis or delay the onset of osteoporosis.

- It can decrease the risk of heart attack by elevating beneficial cholesterol (high density lipoprotein–HDL) levels in the blood.

- It can reduce the likelihood of pelvic organ atrophy by strengthening and supporting the uterus, vagina, bladder, and urinary tract. Pelvic organ atrophy can lead to painful intercourse, urinary urgency, and incontinence.

- It may benefit women with existing musculoskeletal disorders such as rheumatoid arthritis that often worsen after menopause.

ARE THERE DISADVANTAGES TO ESTROGEN REPLACEMENT THERAPY?

The serious disadvantages of estrogen replacement include:

- It increases the risk of breast cancer unless the estrogen estriol is used.

- It increases the risk of uterine cancer unless estrogen is combined with progesterone or the estrogen estriol is used.

- It increases the growth of uterine fibroid tumors.

- It increases the incidence of breast fibroids in women with a personal history of this condition.

- It may increase the risk of gallbladder and liver disease.

- It requires both a financial and a medical commitment due to the cost of the medication and the continuing medical supervision needed.

Other complaints associated with estrogen replacement include: abdominal cramps, amenorrhea, bloating and fluid retention, blood pressure elevation, blood sugar level irregularities, breast tenderness and enlargement, nausea, hair loss, headache, mental depression, vaginal yeast infections, weight gain, a slight increase in incidence of gallstones.

ARE THE SIDE EFFECTS DIFFERENT IF A WOMAN TAKES SYNTHETIC OR NATURAL ESTROGEN?

The side effects of taking estrogen appear to depend on the individual taking it and the strength and type of estrogen she is taking.

Synthetic estrogens are generally stronger and usually cause more side effects. Synthetic estrogens are now used primarily in birth control pills.

It has been reported that women taking estriol, a phytoestrogen (plant derived), do not experience most of the side effects experienced while taking the other forms of estrogen. Estriol appears not to increase cancer risk and may even protect against cancer. However, it is not known if it is protective against osteoporosis.

WHY IS ESTRIOL NOT PRESCRIBED MORE OFTEN?

Estriol is not as strong as the other types of estrogen available for HRT. A stronger dose of estriol (2 to 4 mg) may be required to relieve menopausal discomforts such as hot flashes and vaginal dryness, as opposed to estrone or estradiol (0.6 to 1.25 mg). These higher dosage requirements of estriol sometimes cause stomach upsets in women. Also, studies have not confirmed that estriol has the same benefits to a woman's bone health and cardiovascular system as estrone and estradiol, most commonly prescribed in HRT.

A formulation called tri-estrogen that contains 80% estriol, 10% estrone, and 10% estradiol may be the safest and most effective form of estrogen for women. It is said to provide an adequate dose of estriol to be effective for relieving menopausal discomfort, while the lower percentages of estrone and estradiol are believed to be adequate to benefit the bones and heart.

WHY DOES ESTRIOL HAVE A DIFFERENT EFFECT ON A WOMAN'S BODY THAN ESTRONE AND ESTRADIOL?

Three forms of estrogen are produced naturally by a woman's body: estradiol, estrone, and estriol. Estradiol is the primary estrogen produced by the ovaries, estradiol is converted into estrone by the intestines, and estriol is believed to be produced by a woman's body in connection with progesterone.

Estrone is known to have a stimulating effect on a woman's

breasts and uterine lining. Conjugated estrogens (*Premarin*) are mostly converted to estrone in the intestinal tract. Estriol is believed to have an anticancer effect by blocking the stimulating effects of estrone on breast tissue and the uterine lining.

ARE THERE ADVANTAGES TO TAKING PROGESTIN ALONG WITH ESTROGEN?

Combination estrogen/progestin hormone replacement therapy is most commonly prescribed to women in the U.S. during and after menopause because it has been shown to reduce the risk of uterine cancer that occurs when women take conjugated estrogen alone.

WHAT ARE THE DISADVANTAGES OF ESTROGEN/PROG- ESTIN HORMONE REPLACEMENT THERAPY?

The disadvantages of a combination estrogen/progestin replacement:

- It artificially manipulates the natural menstrual cycle and may cause menstrual periods to continue after menopause, although they are said to diminish over time.
- It may increase the risk of heart disease or stroke.
- Often it is difficult to find a comfortable combination and dosage to make HRT effective in relieving menopausal discomforts, yet eliminate the risks and side effects of both estrogen and progestins.

WHAT ARE THE DISADVANTAGES OF TAKING PROGESTINS?

The negative effects of progestin (synthetic progesterone) replacement:

- It increases the risk of breast cancer.
- It increases the risk of heart disease by decreasing high density lipoprotein (HDL cholesterol) levels.

Common complaints of women taking progestins include abdominal bloating, breast tenderness, fluid retention, headaches, moodiness. However, many of these complaints can be eliminated by reducing progestin dosage.

ARE THE ADVANTAGES AND DISADVANTAGES THE SAME WHETHER A WOMAN TAKES PROGESTIN OR NATURAL PROGESTERONE?

The healthcare practitioners whose patients have used natural progesterone report that most of the side effects associated with synthetic progestins are eliminated. However, women using natural progesterone, just as those taking a progestin, may have a continuation of menstrual periods, or their menstrual periods may return after they have already stopped.

ARE THERE OTHER ADVANTAGES TO USING NATURAL PROGESTERONE?

Natural progesterone has been shown to eliminate many of the discomforts of menopause, such as hot flashes, mood changes, night sweats, and vaginal dryness. It has also been reported that:

- It is a natural diuretic and reduces fluid retention.
- It enhances energy.
- It stimulates thyroid gland function.
- It is a mild antidepressant.

Natural progesterone has been reported to offset more serious health problems by:

- Protecting the breasts from fibrocysts and cancer.
- Reducing the incidence of uterine fibroids (myomas).
- Protecting the uterine lining and prevent endometrial cancer.
- Reducing the risks of osteoporosis by stimulating formation of new bone.
- Normalizing blood clotting.

IS NATURAL PROGESTERONE EFFECTIVE WHEN TAKEN ALONE OR MUST IT BE TAKEN WITH ESTROGEN?

Natural progesterone has been shown to be effective alone or it may be used in conjunction with estrogen. Usually, low doses of natural estrogen such as estriol or tri-estrogen are prescribed for use with natural progesterone.

WHAT ARE THE ADVANTAGES OF TESTOSTERONE IN HRT?

Even while taking estrogen, some women still feel tired and experience a low sex drive. Small dosages of testosterone can eliminate these problems and give a woman an overall feeling of well-being.

DO WOMEN EXPERIENCE SIDE EFFECTS FROM TAKING TESTOSTERONE?

Because testosterone is an androgen (male hormone), naturally manufactured by the ovaries in very small quantities, too high a dosage may result in unwanted hair growth, weight gain, a deeper voice, enlargement of the clitoris, as well as negatively affecting blood cholesterol levels.

DO THE ADVANTAGES AND DISADVANTAGES OF TAKING HRT CHANGE DEPENDING ON HOW LONG A WOMAN TAKES IT?

Some negative side effects of taking *HRT* show up right away. They usually include symptoms that are considered discomforts, rather than health risks. However, the reason most women stop taking *HRT* after a short period of initial use is because it can be difficult to adjust the dosage to a comfortable, effective level.

More serious health risks associated with *HRT* are associated with the length of time it is taken. Depending on a woman's overall health profile and personal risk factors, many doctors may recommend women take *HRT* for a period of four to seven years during menopause to relieve symptoms of discomfort and for a short time after menopause, then stop taking it until later in life, usually around age 60, when the risk of osteoporosis and heart disease is the greatest.

IS THERE ANYTHING A WOMAN CAN DO TO OFFSET THE SIDE EFFECTS OF HRT?

If you experience side effects from *HRT,* your doctor can adjust the dosage to make you more comfortable. It is always best to take the lowest possible effective dosage.

Any adverse effects from *HRT* need to be reported to your doctor. Unusual uterine or vaginal bleeding, breast tenderness, or sensitive masses are considered serious side effects. Report these to your physician immediately.

Various foods, nutritional supplements, herbs, and adjunctive therapies can be helpful, not only to alleviate the discomforts of menopause, but to diminish the side effects of *HRT.* These will be discussed in later chapters.

IF A WOMAN AND HER DOCTOR DECIDE TO ADJUST HER HRT DOSAGE, HOW LONG WILL IT TAKE BEFORE SHE'LL KNOW IF THE NEW DOSAGE IS BETTER FOR HER?

That depends on the individual woman and the side effects she is experiencing. Generally, hormonal adjustments within the body take time. Your doctor can advise you about how long to allow for them.

IF THE SIDE EFFECTS STILL DON'T GO AWAY, WHAT CAN A WOMAN DO?

Many women stop taking *HRT* because, despite dosage adjustments, the side effects are as bad or worse than the natural discomforts of menopause. If that happens, a woman can keep trying other types of hormones or she can decide to discontinue *HRT*.

For women who cannot find the right prescription of *HRT* for their comfort, it might be worthwhile to try the alternative approaches to menopause discussed throughout this book.

CHAPTER 4
▲ ▲ ▲

How Can You Decide If
HRT Is Right for You?

Deciding whether *HRT* is right for you can be confusing and frustrating when your life is already filled with unfamiliar physical and emotional changes. A systematic approach can help you make the *HRT* decision one step at a time.

WHAT STEPS CAN A WOMAN TAKE TO MAKE A DECISION ABOUT HRT?

- First, educate yourself about the pros and cons of hormone replacement therapy.

- Then assess your own health profile, which will show you where the effects and side effects of HRT could be beneficial or detrimental to your health immediately and over the long run.

- Consult a physician and ask for your health to be evaluated with the various laboratory tests and physical examinations detailed in this chapter. Ask for a copy of all your test results to take home and keep in your personal health file.

- Discuss every aspect of your physical condition, your test results, and your treatment choices with your physician. Ask questions. If your questions cannot be answered to your satisfaction, take your test results to another doctor who will answer them.

- Finally, the choice of your own health program is yours alone. You can agree or disagree with any doctor. Their opinions and suggestions can be added to the pool of information you have collected from other sources.

Once you have a total picture of your health and healthcare needs, then you can make an informed decision based on your doctor's opinions, the information you have gathered from your doctor and other sources, and any feelings you have about your own health and medical treatment.

WHO IS A CANDIDATE FOR HRT?

Women who experience extremely debilitating discomfort from hot flashes, heart palpitations, and vaginal dryness during menopause have reported significant relief from *HRT*. Women with a family history of severe osteoporosis or heart disease are being encouraged to take *HRT*.

WHEN IS IT BEST FOR A WOMAN TO AVOID TAKING HRT?

A woman with a family history of cancer is advised to carefully consider her own personal risk factors before deciding to take either estrogen or an estrogen/progestin combination.

Most doctors feel it is not safe for a woman to take estrogen when:

- she has been diagnosed to have or is suspected to have breast cancer,
- she has liver disease,
- she has a blood clotting condition of any kind (thrombophlebitis or thromboembolic disorders).

A woman is advised to evaluate carefully whether the benefits of *HRT* outweigh the potential risks when:

- she has a chronic liver disorder,
- she has substantial excess body weight,
- she has uterine fibroid tumors (myomas),
- she has had a blood clotting disorder (thrombophlebitis or thromboembolism) at any time,
- she has had endometriosis at any time,

- she has had endometrial cancer at any time,
- she has diabetes.

WHAT IF A WOMAN WITH ANY OF THESE CONDITIONS STILL WANTS TO TAKE HRT?

Before any woman decides to take *HRT* it is extremely important that she fully inform her doctor of her entire medical history, especially if she has had any of the conditions listed above.

If you and your doctor agree that *HRT* would be beneficial for you, estriol and natural progesterone may be your safest bet. A monitoring schedule is then very important. A woman who has any of the risk factors listed above needs to be more closely monitored by her physician. Side effects from *HRT* must always be taken seriously by any woman who takes it.

IS A GYNECOLOGIST THE BEST DOCTOR TO CONSULT ABOUT MENOPAUSE AND ITS TREATMENT?

Gynecologists are considered conventional medical specialists in women's healthcare and may be the most helpful to a woman during menopause. Menopausal medicine is quickly emerging as a field of subspecialty in gynecology because the population of women over 45 is increasing.

Still, a woman's healthcare during and after menopause can be furnished by many types of doctors, including primary care physicians, family doctors, endocrinologists, internists, and geriatric specialists in the conventional medical field. In alternative medical fields, a woman may seek treatment from homeopaths, naturopaths, acupuncturists, and chiropractors, as discussed in chapter 5.

HOW CAN YOU AND YOUR DOCTOR DETERMINE IF HRT MIGHT BE BENEFICIAL FOR YOU?

Determining whether *HRT* might be beneficial for any woman requires evaluation by a doctor of the woman's medical records, her medical history, a thorough physical examination, and laboratory testing. Only then can a woman's current overall health status and her potential health risks be evaluated realistically.

WHY ARE A WOMAN'S MEDICAL RECORDS IMPORTANT FOR HER DOCTOR TO HAVE?

Your medical records will communicate your medical history to doctors in clinical terms that will be most useful to them. Often it is not easy for women to remember every detail of their previous health evaluations or medical treatments. You might not be aware of some details or observations made by your previous doctors that are contained in your medical records.

WHERE DO YOUR MEDICAL RECORDS COME FROM?

If you keep a personal file of your past medical records, share it with your doctor. If you do not, be prepared to give your doctor the names, addresses, and telephone numbers of your previous physicians so your past medical records can be obtained. You will need to sign a form giving your doctor permission to ask for your records from another doctor or a laboratory.

WHAT DOES YOUR DOCTOR NEED TO KNOW ABOUT YOUR HEALTH?

Your doctor will want to know about your personal and family medical history, what medical treatments you are currently receiving, and any current symptoms and the length of time you have been experiencing them. These will indicate what medical conditions you may currently have, whether menopause is a possibility for you, and if it is, what stage of menopause you may have reached.

WHY DOES YOUR DOCTOR NEED TO KNOW YOUR FAMILY MEDICAL HISTORY?

The entire medical history of you and your family are important when considering *HRT.* Genetic predisposition to certain disorders and diseases, such as breast cancer, uterine cancer, heart disease, osteoporosis, and diabetes may make it risky or even dangerous for some women to undergo *HRT.* (These conditions will be addressed in chapters 9 through 12.)

WHAT DOES YOUR DOCTOR NEED TO KNOW ABOUT YOUR CURRENT HEALTH?

Your doctor will need to know:

- about any medical treatment you are currently receiving,
- your current and recent physical complaints and symptoms,
- what medications you are currently taking (including over-the-counter pain relievers, antacids, and cold remedies) or have taken in the past,
- any nutritional supplements, herbs, and nondrug remedies you have recently or are currently taking,
- your diet, lifestyle, and sexual habits.

You must be completely honest with your doctor so that a realistic treatment program can be suggested and discussed with you. Make notes ahead of time of your medications and supplements, physical complaints, and symptoms. While no complaint or symptom is too incidental, heart palpitations and bone discomfort are especially important. Take your notes with you to the doctor's office, because sometimes it is difficult to remember everything you want to tell the doctor once you're there.

Based on this information, your doctor will conduct a complete physical examination to determine your overall health status and risk factors. If menopause is a factor in your healthcare, your doctor can evaluate the hormone levels and production in your body during your physical exam and after a variety of laboratory tests.

WHAT CAN YOU EXPECT DURING A DOCTOR'S PHYSICAL EXAMINATION OF YOU?

You need a complete general physical examination so your

doctor can assess your overall health and suggest appropriate treatments. The exam will include:

- a blood pressure reading to see if your heart is pumping blood at a normal rate (an indication of your cardiovascular health),
- a gynecological and pelvic exam for signs of menopause or abnormality, when your doctor will
  - look at the color and condition of your vaginal lining
  - look at the condition, shape, and position of your cervix
  - feel the shape and size of your uterus to determine if it contains growths or irregularities
  - feel your ovaries to determine if they are of normal size and shape
- a pap smear will be taken and sent to a laboratory to determine
  - if cervical cells are normal
  - a maturation index, indicating the estrogen effect in your vagina. (This will be explained fully in chapter 12.)

WHAT OTHER LABORATORY TESTS WILL BE NEEDED?

The following laboratory tests are also important:

- Urinalysis. You will be asked to give a sample of your urine to be sent to a laboratory for analysis to determine that you are not pregnant, and insure that your kidneys, bladder, and liver are functioning properly and are free of infection.
- Blood will be drawn and sent to a laboratory for
  - a complete blood count to determine if you have a healthy number of red and white blood cells, which will show among other things if you have developed anemia from excessive menstrual bleeding.
  - a blood chemistry test to analyze the chemicals in your blood, which will show if you have normal levels of

minerals and other elements in your blood, giving your doctor an idea of your overall health.

- an analysis of your blood clotting factors, especially important if you have a personal or family history of blood-clotting disorders or disease.

- a cholesterol count to determine if your levels are normal, an indication of cardiovascular health and heart disease risk. Make sure your cholesterol count includes total cholesterol, HDL, LDL, and triglyceride levels.

- fasting blood sugar levels if you have a personal or family history of diabetes or hypoglycemia.

- a kidney function test.

- a liver function test, important if you are considering HRT in pill form, because the hormones will pass through the liver before entering your circulation.

- a thyroid function test because HRT effectiveness in your body can be affected by thyroid function and your thyroid function can be affected by HRT.

- a test for syphilis and possibly HIV (human immunodeficiency virus).

- Progesterone challenge or endometrial biopsy may be needed if you have a personal history of endometriosis or irregular uterine bleeding.

Your doctor may also ask you to see a radiologist for additional health evaluation.

WHAT DOES A RADIOLOGIST DO?

A radiologist uses advanced medical detection machines to assess the condition of your breasts, pelvic organs, and bones with these tests

- Mammogram. You may be sent for a mammogram to determine if your breast tissue is normal and healthy. The results will also be compared to your baseline mammogram if you had one previously. If you have not, this one will become your baseline for future comparisons.

A mammogram is especially important if you have a personal or family history of breast irregularities or cancer.

- Bone Scan. May be appropriate if you have had bone discomfort, fractures, or a personal or family history of osteoporosis. It will be compared to your baseline if you have had previous bone scans or become your baseline for future scans.

- Pelvic Ultrasound. You may need this noninvasive test to detect abnormalities of your uterus, endometrium (lining of the uterus), or ovaries.

- Electrocardiogram. While not normally suggested for women at menopause, if you are having heart palpitations with hot flashes or without them, emphasize that to your doctor and discuss your need for an EKG. This may be more important if your family has a history of cardiovascular disease and heart attacks at an early age.

WHAT TESTS CAN A DOCTOR DO TO DETERMINE THE AMOUNT OF HORMONES YOUR BODY IS PRODUCING?

- Maturation index of cells taken from your vaginal lining similar to a Pap smear of the cervix will indicate the effect of estrogen on your vaginal tissues.

The quantity of three types of vaginal cells are observed under a microscope: superficial cells, parabasal cells, and basal cells. A majority of parabasal cells usually indicates little stimulation of the vaginal tissue by estrogen and usually means menopause. (A maturation index is fully explained in chapter 12.)

- Sampling your blood in a laboratory can measure your levels of hormones. If the estrogen level in a woman's blood is low it may indicate menopause, especially when the FSH (follicle-stimulating hormone) level is high.

WHAT IS FSH?

FSH is a hormone released by the hypothalamus and pituitary

glands of the brain in the complicated interaction between them and the ovaries. FSH and LH (luteinizing hormone) stimulate the ovarian follicles to ripen and release eggs. When ovarian follicles cannot produce enough estrogen to release an egg, a message is sent to the hypothalamus and pituitary glands. They, in turn, release more FSH, sending a return message to stimulate the ovaries into producing estrogen. When the ovaries are not able to produce enough estrogen to release an egg, the FSH level in the blood will be high and estrogen levels low, usually indicating menopause.

HOW WILL YOU LEARN THE RESULTS OF ALL OF YOUR TESTS?

Your doctor will call you and discuss your test results over the phone or suggest you return to the office for another consultation. Do not be shy about asking questions about your test results at this time or about calling the doctor later with follow-up questions.

WILL THE DOCTOR GIVE YOU A COPY OF YOUR TEST RESULTS?

Few doctors offer to do that. However, you are entitled to have copies of your test results. It is a good idea to keep a copy of them at home in your own personal health file.

HOW DOES THE AMOUNT OF HORMONE PRODUCTION IN A WOMAN'S BODY INFLUENCE A DOCTOR'S RECOMMENDATION FOR HRT?

A woman still producing hormones, even low levels of estrogen and progesterone, who is not experiencing any significant discomfort associated with menopause, such as hot flashes, heart palpitations, or vaginal dryness, is usually not advised to start *HRT,* unless she is at extreme risk for heart disease or osteoporosis.

WHAT MONITORING PROGRAM IS BEST WHILE YOU TAKE HRT?

Every woman undergoing *HRT* needs regular medical check-ups and routine monitoring semiannually and annually, including Semi-annual tests and examinations:

- blood pressure reading
- red blood cell count (hemoglobin)
- blood cholesterol screening, if she has a personal history of high cholesterol or a family history of heart disease
- clinical breast examination by her physician
- urinalysis

Annual Tests and Examinations:

- pelvic and rectal exam
- pap smear, if she has an intact uterus
- mammogram, annually for women over 50 or for women over 40 who are at high risk for breast cancer. Current American Cancer Society guidelines suggest a mammogram for women between 40 and 49 every year or two, depending on their personal medical history and risk factors.

A complete general physical exam is advised at appropriate intervals if you take *HRT*, including an EKG (electrocardiogram) for women at high risk for heart disease and a bone scan for women at high risk for osteoporosis.

HOW LONG WILL YOU NEED TO TAKE HRT*?*

Every woman can make this choice based on her personal health profile, risk factors, and her success with *HRT*. Many women who decide to take *HRT* and experience benefits from it stay on it for the rest of their lives. Some women take it only during menopause and for a short time after. Others take it during menopause, stop, and begin again after age 60 when the incidence of heart attack in women increases dramatically. The average age of first heart attacks in women is 74 and of hip fractures, 80.

WHAT IF YOU START TAKING HRT AND HAVE SIDE EFFECTS?

Report any side effects while taking *HRT* to your doctor immediately, especially breast changes or abnormal bleeding. Depending on your symptoms and their severity, your doctor may change your prescription to different types or brands of hormones, prescribe lower doses, or you may elect to discontinue *HRT* altogether.

To avoid side effects from *HRT,* it is better to take the lowest effective dosages available to you.

HOW MANY WOMEN TAKE HRT DURING AND AFTER MENOPAUSE?

Approximately 50 percent of all menopausal women take *HRT* for some period of time.

HOW MANY WOMEN CONTINUE HRT?

About half of those who start *HRT* continue it.

WHY DO WOMEN STOP HRT?

Many women say they stop *HRT* because the side effects are more uncomfortable than the menopausal discomfort they experience without *HRT.* Others may stop taking it on the advice of their physicians following menopause after considering their risk factors for serious health problems.

HOW DO YOU KNOW IF YOU SHOULD STOP?

Adjusting dosage to eliminate side effects seems to be the biggest problem for women who stop *HRT.* Once a comfortable dose is found, it will still take time for the effects of the medication to benefit your overall health.

HOW CAN YOU TELL IF IT'S WORKING?

If *HRT* is working for you, it will alleviate discomfort during menopause. After that, lab tests can determine if *HRT* is beneficial for your bones, your heart, and your uterus. Follow-up testing is a routine every woman who takes *HRT* should expect.

WHAT HAPPENS IF YOU DECIDE TO STOP TAKING HRT?

If you decided to take *HRT* and experienced side effects after only a short time of usage, it is possible to just stop. However, if you have been taking *HRT* for an extended period, it is better to wean yourself gradually from the drugs by reducing dosages. You should discuss that with your physician, who may recommend skipping either days or weeks. Your doctor may also suggest it is better to systematically lower your prescription dosage over time before you skip days.

WHAT WILL THE EFFECTS BE ON YOUR BODY AFTER YOU STOP?

You could experience the physical discomforts of menopause if your body has never been given the opportunity to make its own natural hormonal adjustments at the time of your menopause. Further, an estrogen-supplemented body may lose bone mass during the few years immediately following withdrawal from estrogen.

HOW CAN YOU OFFSET THE SIDE EFFECTS OF ESTROGEN WITHDRAWAL WHEN YOU STOP HRT?

Try following the advice given to most women at menopause: consume a well-balanced, nutritious diet and eliminate detrimental food intake, supplementing your diet with vitamins and minerals or herbs if you choose; adjust your lifestyle to include regular, routine weight-bearing exercise for your bones, and devise ways to reduce stress and relax. Finally, continue to monitor your health and get regular medical examinations.

CHAPTER 5

▲ ▲ ▲

Can HRT and Non-Drug Treatments Work Together During Menopause?

American women are now incorporating non-drug medical treatments into their healthcare programs because they understand, as do their conventional medical doctors, that drugs are not the only answer for a woman during menopause. Diet, lifestyle changes, and non-drug therapies have been proven for centuries throughout the world to benefit a woman's overall health, even enhancing the effectiveness of conventional medical treatment during menopause and into the later years.

WHAT'S THE DIFFERENCE BETWEEN CONVENTIONAL MEDICINE AND NON-DRUG MEDICAL TREATMENT OF MENOPAUSE?

Conventional and alternative medicine have the same goal: to relieve a woman's discomfort during the transitional years of menopause and help her to achieve optimal health during menopause and into her later years of life. The differences between conventional and alternative medicine begin with their approaches.

HOW DOES CONVENTIONAL MEDICINE APPROACH THE TREATMENT OF MENOPAUSE?

Conventional medicine often considers menopause as a hormone-deficiency disorder and attempts to correct the imbalances that develop within a woman's hormonal system during and after menopause. Using *HRT* to restore a woman's hormone balance to that similar to her premenopausal years has been shown to alleviate the discomforts of menopause and to offset some of the serious health problems women may develop in their later years.

HOW DOES ALTERNATIVE MEDICINE APPROACH THE TREATMENT OF MENOPAUSE?

The alternative medical approach focuses on strengthening the female body by encouraging it to balance, regulate, and normalize itself during the transition to menopause. Alternative treatments during menopause usually favor non-drug therapies.

WHICH IS BETTER?

Conventional medicine and non-drug therapies each have a place in the treatment of menopause because every woman is unique in body, mind, and beliefs about how she chooses to handle her own health. Arguments can be made for and against any treatment program.

Conventional medical treatments using *HRT* are attractive to some women because they seem easier and more convenient, requiring less attention to daily health maintenance. But *HRT* can have side effects and because conventional medical treatment is usually considered interventionist, some experts believe that it short-circuits the natural healing and balancing abilities of the body.

Alternative medical treatments don't always show the immediate results women experience with *HRT.* Non-drug therapies usually require a greater commitment by the individual woman to her own daily health care. Diet and lifestyle factors will be considered more seriously by physicians who embrace alternative methods, even those who combine alternative approaches with conventional medicine.

DO WOMEN GET BETTER RESULTS WITH CONVENTIONAL MEDICINE OR ALTERNATIVES?

That depends on the individual. Whatever their treatment of choice, the women who seem to do best during and after menopause are those who take more responsibility for their own health and well being, and who understand that menopause is a natural transition of the female body from one stage of life to another.

WHAT DOES CONVENTIONAL MEDICINE PROPOSE FOR THE TREATMENT OF MENOPAUSE?

HRT has been shown to alleviate the discomforts some women experience during menopause—among them hot flashes, night sweats, heart palpitations, and vaginal dryness. While *HRT* is also prescribed to offset higher risks of osteoporosis, heart disease, and pelvic organ disorders that some women experience after menopause, there can be side effects. These health risks associated with *HRT* include increased incidence of uterine and breast cancer in some women.

Conventional medicine also recognizes the importance of diet and nutrition, exercise, stress reduction, and eliminating smoking for women, especially during the menopausal years and later.

HOW DOES ALTERNATIVE TREATMENT DIFFER?

An alternative, non-drug approach during menopause and into later life shifts the emphasis from *HRT* to natural ways of encouraging the body to balance and heal itself. The focus on dietary, nutritional, and lifestyle changes is very important and may be supported by acupuncture, herbs, and homeopathic remedies that have been shown to be effective.

Specific dietary and nutritional changes with nutritional and herbal supplements have been shown to alleviate the discomforts of menopause: hot flashes, night sweats, heart palpitations, and vaginal dryness, as well as to reduce the risk of osteoporosis and heart disease. Natural non-drug therapies avoid side effects and the risks of prescription hormone replacement.

CAN YOU USE BOTH CONVENTIONAL AND ALTERNATIVE MEDICAL TREATMENTS DURING AND AFTER MENOPAUSE?

Clinical evaluation of a woman's health status provided by conventional medicine can be important during and after menopause, because this is the scientific evidence any woman needs before she embarks on a treatment program of any kind. The tests provide a baseline against which she can gauge her ongoing health status and progress as she ages.

This evidence is usually provided by clinical tests performed by or requested by gynecologists, endocrinologists, and radiologists. Gynecologists are conventional women's healthcare experts. Endocrinologists are experts in glandular and hormonal functions of the body. Radiologists conduct examinations with technical medical machinery and evaluate the results.

Some doctors are educated in both conventional medicine and the alternative therapies. These physicians can produce a woman's scientific health profile and then offer suggestions for both conventional and alternative treatments.

Seeking assistance from both a conventional doctor and an alternative healthcare provider may seem like an added expense, but it can benefit some women by providing the best of both approaches.

Many women choose to have their primary care directed by either a conventional doctor or an alternative healthcare provider, following the advice and treatment by the other as adjunctive treatment.

HOW DO ALTERNATIVE TREATMENTS AFFECT HRT?

Alternative treatments have been shown to enhance the effects of *HRT* by reducing dosage requirements, thus alleviating the health risks associated with *HRT* or even eliminating some side effects.

Non-drug treatments of menopause have been shown in some women to eliminate the need for *HRT* altogether.

WHAT ARE SOME NON-DRUG APPROACHES FOR TREATING MENOPAUSE?

There are various methods for treating menopause in conjunction with *HRT*, or without it: acupressure and acupuncture, aromatherapy, Ayurveda, Chinese medicine, chiropractic, homeopathic medicine, and naturopathic medicine.

An overview of these adjunctive therapies and their benefits during menopause follows. For more information, see the Suggested Reading List and Resources section.

ACUPRESSURE AND ACUPUNCTURE

WHAT ARE ACUPRESSURE AND ACUPUNCTURE?

Acupressure and acupuncture are painless, non-toxic methods of natural healing used from ancient times in the Orient.

In a series of treatments, they redirect and restore energy flow in a complex system of pathways through the body by stimulating meridian points that are connected to specific organs and bodily functions. It is believed that when the energy flow through the body is obstructed or out of balance, disease or illness results and the body cannot naturally heal itself.

HOW IS ACUPRESSURE APPLIED TO THE BODY?

Acupressure can be properly applied by a licensed massage therapist or chiropractor who either massages or strokes the body to restore energy flow or applies finger pressure on specific points of the body.

Many books on the market show women how to apply acupressure on themselves.

HOW CAN ACUPRESSURE HELP A WOMAN DURING MENOPAUSE?

Pressure applied to specific points on the hands and feet can help stimulate the ovaries, uterus, and adrenal, pituitary, thyroid, and parathyroid glands to balance hormone production and reduce hot flashes. Profuse or prolonged menstruation can be controlled by applying pressure to the insides of both legs, five inches below the knees.

HOW IS ACUPUNCTURE APPLIED TO THE BODY?

Acupuncture is performed by a licensed acupuncturist who inserts hair-thin needles into specific points on the body to release energy blocks or to direct and rechannel energy. Sometimes electrodes are attached to the needles for more stimulation. Healing herbs may also be burned in the room during treatments.

HOW CAN ACUPUNCTURE HELP A WOMAN DURING MENOPAUSE?

Besides releasing energy blocks and rechanneling energy, the needles can also stimulate the release of pain relieving endorphines by the body. Acupuncture provides a feeling of improved vitality and well-being while encouraging the body to balance and heal itself.

AROMATHERAPY

WHAT IS AROMATHERAPY?

Aromatherapy, related to the ancient science of herbal medicine, uses aromatic essential oils from plants to assist in physical healing of the body by restoring energy balance, promoting cell regeneration, eliminating toxins from the body, and calming, soothing, and elevating the emotions.

WHERE DO THE AROMATHERAPY OILS COME FROM?

The oils are non-oily fluids condensed from various parts of herbs and flowers.

HOW IS AROMATHERAPY USED?

Aromatherapy oils easily penetrate the skin and are added to bath water, massage oils, or compresses. They may also be dispersed in steam, inhalers, or air diffusers.

Because these essential oils are herbs in very concentrated form, to avoid irritation or a hypersensitive reaction, aromatherapy oils should not be applied directly to the skin undiluted or near the eyes, mouth, nose, or genitals. If irritation results from the use of a specific oil, discontinue it. Always keep essential oils out of the reach of children.

Essential oils can be taken internally, but a toxic reaction is possible. Therefore, follow the advice of an herbalist before ingesting essential oils.

HOW CAN AROMATHERAPY BENEFIT WOMEN DURING MENOPAUSE?

Because of the growing popularity of aromatherapy, many magazine articles and books are available detailing the uses of individual herbal essences. The following herbs have been found to be helpful as aromatherapy during menopause:

- Basil alleviates fatigue.
- Chamomile and lavender in combination improve relaxation and calm nerves.
- Cypress, geranium, or rose ease heavy periods.
- Juniper, lavender, or rosemary easy muscle and joint pain.
- Lavender or peppermint ease headaches.
- Lemongrass or ylang-ylang ease PMS.
- Neroli or lavender alleviate insomnia.
- Sage eases tension and depression and balances hormones.
- Thyme alleviates insomnia and improves circulation.

Herbal combinations can be more effective than using herbs individually. In bath water combine three drops of each oil: basil and cypress, thyme or rosemary, or rosemary and basil.

Add to almond or olive oil for massage three drops of each oil: thyme, rosemary, basil, and cypress.

AYURVEDA

WHAT IS AYURVEDA?

Ayurveda is a medical system practiced in India for over 4,000 years, and still used today to improve the quality of life and for longevity. Specific diets, natural therapies, music, herbs, and aromatherapy are used to balance the body's energy and improve its ability to heal itself.

The exact medical program for an individual woman is determined after considering her physical and psychological body type. A daily and seasonal lifestyle and behavior routine is suggested to help an individual integrate with nature's biological rhythms. Specific diets are based on an individual's body type and imbalances. And herbal preparations are selected from thousands used over the centuries.

HOW CAN AYURVEDA BENEFIT WOMEN DURING MENOPAUSE?

Ayurveda can be effective for relieving the discomforts of menopause with dietary changes and the use of medicinal herbs. Over the long run, Ayurvedic changes in diet and lifestyle can lead to a healthier, more balanced body and mind.

CHINESE MEDICINE

WHAT IS TRADITIONAL CHINESE MEDICINE?

Chinese medicine has been practiced for as long as 5,000 years. Its underlying theme is that a healthy person is one who is harmonious and in balance. When disharmony results in physical and psychological disease, it is necessary to rebalance the person by using acupuncture, Chinese herbs, and by making dietary adjustments.

HOW DOES TRADITIONAL CHINESE MEDICINE VIEW MENOPAUSE?

Traditional Chinese medicine considers blood to be the material foundation of the body and the mind. Blood is stored in the liver, generated by the spleen, propelled by the heart, and supplied to the bones, marrow, and tissues by the kidneys.

The kidneys govern reproductive function. Sufficient energy in a woman's kidneys is necessary for fertility, libido, regeneration of the entire body, and tissue elasticity and strength.

At puberty, a woman's kidney energy increases, sending excess blood to the uterus. During her reproductive years, the kidneys supply enough blood for fertility, but as a woman matures, the blood flow from her kidneys diminishes, leading to menopause.

Although menopause is considered a natural cycle in a woman's life and can be experienced without discomfort, problems occur when kidney energy is depleted and cannot sustain the rest of the body. That is when the discomfort of menopause occurs and deterioration of health begins.

HOW CAN TRADITIONAL CHINESE MEDICINE BENEFIT A WOMAN DURING MENOPAUSE?

For a smooth transition through menopause, acupuncture, dietary adjustments, and Chinese herbs are used to nourish and strengthen a woman's kidney essence as it affects her other organs. Hot flashes and anxiety are considered a weakness of the heart; irregular menstrual flow and irritability a weakness of the liver; heavy menstrual bleeding and food cravings a weakness of the spleen. Chinese herbs commonly used include:

- Bao shao yao for thinning hair
- Chi shao yao and Di fu zi for dry, itchy skin
- Fo ti, an endocrine system tonic, rejuvenates, strengthens, and energizes.
- Nuo dao gen for night sweats
- Qing huo for hot flashes

- Sang shen zi for thinning hair
- She chaung zi and Tu fu ling for sore, dry vagina

There are also Chinese herbal combination formulas available as tea in health food stores. These medicinals have names such as: American Ginseng, Relaxing, Ultra Slim, Sugar-Bal, etc. with corresponding aspects clearly written on the tea packaging. Because these herbal combinations can have a powerful effect on the body, it is best to read the information provided in the packaging and follow instructions. Start slow and be aware of your body's reactions.

CHIROPRACTIC MEDICINE

WHAT IS CHIROPRACTIC MEDICINE?

Chiropractic medicine is based on manipulation of the spine and joints and has been an integral part of healing throughout recorded history. Many chiropractic healing programs also incorporate exercise and diet, acupuncture, massage, homeopathy, and kine- siology, a system of muscle testing that reveals organ malfunctions through weakness of the related muscles of the body.

HOW CAN CHIROPRACTIC MEDICINE BENEFIT A WOMAN DURING MENOPAUSE?

Chiropractic medicine helps restore the body's ability to heal and balance itself by relieving pressure on the spinal nerve roots that control energy flow throughout the body. The adjunctive therapies used in chiropractic medicine can also help relieve the discomforts of menopause and assist the body in strengthening and supporting itself into the later years.

HERBS

HOW ARE HERBS USED IN HEALTH CARE?

The wide range of medicinal uses of herbs is well documented throughout history. Because herbs come from a living source and have all the nutrients of concentrated foods, they can nourish and balance the body, enabling it to heal and regulate itself.

While drugs and chemicals treat the symptoms of a physical problem, herbs are assimilated by the body as nourishment and find their way to the source of the problem. Therefore, results may not be seen as quickly with herbs as with drugs. But over time, the healing effects of herbs can restore the body to optimal health through renewal and regeneration by reversing the problem.

Even though immediate improvement can be seen within days of taking herbs, chronic health problems will take longer to heal. It is said that natural healing takes one month for every year the problem existed.

ARE THERE SIDE EFFECTS FROM TAKING HERBS?

Most herbs, as edible plants, are safe to take in small quantities as natural medicines. Occasionally, as with a specific food, an individual may have a mild allergy-type reaction to certain herbs. The key to avoiding an adverse reaction is moderation, both in formulation and in dosage. Anything taken in excess can cause negative side effects.

Because some herbs can have a powerful effect in your body, it is best to consult a healthcare professional who has been trained in the use of herbs before you take them.

ARE HERBS TAKEN INDIVIDUALLY OR IN COMBINATION?

Generally, herbs are said to work better when taken in combinations for several reasons:

- each formula compound contains two to five primary agent herbs that are part of the blend for specific purposes. Since all body parts and most disease symptoms are interrelated, it is better to use an herbal combination that will affect each part of your problem.
- a combination lets you include herbs that can work at different stages of healing within your body.

- a combination of several herbs with similar properties can increase the effectiveness of each herb.
- no two people or their bodies are alike.
- finally, some very potent herbs should not be used alone but are beneficial in small amounts in combinations because they act as catalysts.

HOW LONG ARE HERBS TAKEN?

Herbs taken for medicinal purposes work best when taken only as long as symptoms occur. Within a week or so an herb will usually do its job within the body. If the symptoms return, a woman may be advised to begin taking the herbs again.

Herbs for nutritional purposes can be taken over longer periods of time.

HOW CAN A WOMAN KNOW WHAT HERBS TO TAKE?

Deciding which herbs would most benefit your individual health needs may be difficult because herbs can have several types of effects in the body. They break up toxins, cleanse, nourish, tone, and lubricate, freeing the body to heal itself.

Numerous books on the market describe various herbs and their medicinal and nutritional uses, but if you embark on a healing program, natural or not, it is always best to consult an expert. Herbal therapies can be recommended by herbalists and are used in acupuncture, Ayurveda, Chinese medicine, chiropractic care, homeopathy, and naturopathy.

HOW ARE HERBS TAKEN?

Herbs can be taken as tea, tablets, capsules, and extracts. They can be used as a douche for vaginal infections, applied topically in compresses, mixed with creams for application on the skin, or added to bathwater.

WHAT SPECIFIC HERBS CAN BENEFIT A WOMAN DURING MENOPAUSE?

Some herbs have been shown to be beneficial for women during and after menopause even without taking HRT. While taking HRT, some herbs may enhance its effectiveness and result in lower dosage requirements or they may alleviate side effects. Because herbs can have powerful effects and side effects, it is best to consult an herbalist or holistic practitioner before using herbs for medicinal purposes. A healthcare professional may suggest taking the following herbs:

- Alfalfa promotes estrogen production in the body. It is also an excellent source of minerals, vitamins and chlorophyll. Its calcium content benefits bones.
- Anise has an estrogenic effect.
- Astragalus enhances energy and the immune system.
- Avena (oats) helps balance hormones, nourish nerves and adrenal glands, enhancing energy. Weekly intake of Avena rejuvenates bones, skin and hair, nerves and sexual sensitivity.
- Beth Root helps alleviate irregular periods, heavy periods and breakthrough bleeding.
- Black Cohosh contains estrogenic substances. It lowers blood pressure, regulates menstruation, eases ovarian or uterine pain of menstruation, and alleviates nervous conditions. It is especially beneficial for women with hypoglycemia who have been shown to experience more discomfort during menopause. If you get a headache while taking black cohosh, you may also need a progestational herb, such as sarsaparilla or Mexican yam.
- Blessed Thistle assists in hormone balancing, soothes nerves, improves memory, calms, and helps alleviate depression and lethargy.
- Bupleurum relieves constrictions in the body.
- Burdock Root encourages the body to produce estrogen. It is a tonic and an aphrodisiac.
- Chamomile soothes nerves and relaxes.

- Cascara Sagrada helps to alleviate constipation.
- Catnip relaxes and calms.
- Cayenne taken daily in capsules or 1/4 teaspoon mixed in water or juice increases energy as a tonic for circulation and the heart.
- Celery Seed soothes nerves and relaxes; helps alleviate incontinence.
- Chasteberry (Vitex), containing both estrogen- and progesterone-like compounds, regulates progesterone in relation to estrogen, promoting hormone balance. It is considered one of the most effective herbs for alleviating menopausal discomforts, including night sweats and hot flashes.
- Chickweed eaten in a salad, as tea, or in capsules can alleviate constipation.
- Clove added in small amounts to other teas will enhance their aspects.
- Crampbark eases painful, heavy periods.
- Damiana assists in balancing hormones. It is a mild aphrodisiac, soothes the nerves, helps alleviate depression, and increases energy.
- Dandelion Root helps alleviate constipation and helps to regulate blood sugar. Dandelion flowers and leaves made into tea will soothe the nerves.
- Dill reduces estrogen production.
- Dong Quai (angelica), sometimes called the female ginseng, is often suggested to women during menopause because it is an estrogen balancer. It strengthens and tones the overall body, increases energy, lowers blood pressure, and helps to alleviate hot flashes and vaginal dryness. Because it contains vitamin B-12 and folic acid, it may prevent anemia caused by excessive menstrual bleeding, but should not be taken during excessive menstrual flow. Its iron and vitamin E content rebuilds blood. However, some women have found that taking dong quai makes them feel nervous, similar to PMS. These women are advised to take black cohosh instead.

- Evening Primrose Oil aids hormone balancing and reduces inflammation in the uterine cavity.
- False Unicorn Root tones the reproductive organs, aids in hormone balancing, helps relieve depression and cramps, and is an aphrodisiac.
- Fennel soothes the stomach and benefits the liver.
- Ginger warms and stimulates, but can promote bleeding.
- Ginkgo improves circulation, increases oxygen supply to brain, and enhances memory.
- Gotu Kola enhances energy and stamina and promotes longevity by improving memory and preventing senility.
- Horsetail (Shavegrass) contains an easily absorbed form of silicon, which improves calcium absorption, strengthens bones, and contributes to the production of collagen, making it beneficial to connective tissue, skin, hair, and nails. Its iron and vitamin E content rebuilds blood.
- Kelp (and other seaweeds) taken daily in capsules or used as a salt substitute soothes nerves and nourishes thyroid and adrenal glands, preventing fatigue and alleviating many menopausal symptoms. It strengthens the urinary tract and is beneficial for the brain. Kelp is an excellent source of vitamins and minerals, including calcium to benefit bones and silicon to benefit skin.
- Lady's Slipper can relieve anxiety and insomnia.
- Licorice Root contains the compound estriol, and is generally beneficial for women during menopause. It contains cortisone-like elements, restores and stimulates adrenal glands, enhances energy, and assists in stabilizing blood sugar. However, it should not be taken when high blood pressure or hyperadrenal conditions exist. It needs to be used with awareness of your body's reactions.
- Motherwort is reported to help early menopausal problems, including irregular menstrual cycles, clotted blood flow, and hot flashes. It soothes nerves. Because it can induce uterine bleeding, motherwort should not be taken when pregnant or when menstrual periods are heavy.

- Nettle leaves cooked as greens or taken as tea or juice nourish the endocrine system, especially the adrenal glands, reduce fatigue, slow heavy menstrual flow, and alleviate constipation. They are also an excellent source of necessary vitamins and minerals.
- Oregon Grape Root may alleviate chronic constipation when taken daily as a decoction or tincture. It is beneficial for kidneys.
- Passion Flower calms the mind and body, making it useful for anxiety, insomnia, depression, and migraine headaches.
- Pau d'Arco soothes the nerves, calms, and helps alleviate depression, irritability, and lethargy.
- Peppermint and spearmint are calming and soothing.
- Red Raspberry leaf, a tonic for the uterus and mucous membranes, relieves lower body discomfort, cramps, and helps control frequent or excessive bleeding.
- Sage promotes estrogen production. Reduces sweating, easing hot flashes.
- St. John's Wart alleviates insomnia, depression and lethargy, poor memory, and hypertension.
- Sarsaparilla promotes progesterone and testosterone production in the body. It is frequently used by women in England to relieve discomforts of PMS and menopause. Combined with Siberian Ginseng, it increases energy and is an aphrodisiac.
- Saw Palmetto Berries are a reproductive organ tonic.
- Senna promotes bowel regularity and should not be taken by anyone with serious intestinal problems.
- Skullcap calms and repairs nerves, relieves ovarian or uterine pain, and subdues excessive sex drive.
- Siberian Ginseng is regarded as a toning and vitalizing herb fr reproductive glands and may be helpful during menopause. It soothes nerves, calms, and helps alleviate depression, irritability, and lethargy. It also increases energy and stamina and assists in hormone balancing. However, one problem with ginseng is that the variety and quality of the herb available in the United States is inconsistent. Some women find it too stimulating, adding to their nervousness and irritability during menopause.

Dong Quai may be a better choice for these women.

- Squaw Vine is a uterine and ovarian tonic. It eases menstrual irregularities.
- Strawberry Leaf eases heavy, painful periods.
- Suma encourages estrogen production in the body, enhances oxygen flow to body cells, and is a tonic.
- Thyme reduces estrogen production.
- Valerian Root calms and soothes.
- Vervain eases emotional upsets and anxiety.
- Wild Yam Root increases production of female hormones. It eases uterine and ovarian pain, and heavy, painful periods.
- Yerba Mate increases energy and stamina, and alleviates constipation and lethargy.

Numerous herbal combinations on the market are formulated for women during menopause:

- To balance estrogen: angelica, false unicorn, dong quai, wild yam, or licorice root for estrogen. Caution: licorice may raise blood pressure.
- To help hot flashes: sarsaparilla and ginseng tea.
- For heavy menstruation and breakthrough bleeding: shepherd's purse or nettles, with alfalfa. Good sources for vitamin K.
- For relaxation: raspberry, lime blossom, and pulsatilla.
- An herbal formula used by Amish women during menopause, called Lydia Pinkham's Remedy, contains: licorice, camomile, pleurisy root, Jamaica dogwood, black cohosh, life plane, and dandelion root.

HOMEOPATHY

WHAT IS HOMEOPATHY?

Homeopathy was developed by a German physician in the early 1800s. Since then it has been used extensively throughout the world, especially in Australia, Europe, India, and South America. The medical philosophy of homeopathy is that disease ia an imbalance of energy or disturbance of vital forces of the body. Homeopathy believes the body can restore its own balance and its symptoms are expressions of the body trying to rebalance itself. The homeopathic physician uses your symptoms as signposts to determine what imbalances your body is trying to correct and then selects the precise homeopathic remedy to assist the body in the natural healing process.

HOW DOES HOMEOPATHIC MEDICINE DIFFER FROM CONVENTIONAL MEDICINE?

Drugs used in conventional medicine, usually made from chemicals or synthetic modifications of natural substances, are designed to eliminate symptoms, not the cause of the symptoms.

Homeopathic remedies, regulated by the FDA since the turn of the century, are considered safe to be sold over-the-counter without a prescription. They are made from naturally occurring substances of plants, earth minerals, or animal sources and are designed to stimulate and increase the ability of the body to heal itself.

HOW DO HOMEOPATHIC REMEDIES WORK?

The basic principle of homeopathic remedies is similar to vaccination, although the active ingredients of homeopathic remedies are all natural. A tiny amount of the active ingredient in a homeopathic remedy is recognized by the body as an intruder. In response, the body's natural abilities to eliminate the intruder are activated, so selecting the exact remedies for a particular individual is important.

HOW LONG ARE HOMEOPATHIC REMEDIES TAKEN?

Homeopathic remedies work on the theory that less is better. So small doses over a limited period of time usually show results. As soon as symptoms start to improve, discontinue use of the remedy. A series of different remedies may be needed over a longer period of time as the relief of one symptom may reveal another symptom while the body goes through its natural healing process.

HOW ARE HOMEOPATHIC REMEDIES TAKEN?

Homeopathic remedies are taken either in liquid form or in tablets placed under the tongue. The remedy enters your bloodstream directly through the mucous membranes of the mouth. Fifteen minutes before and after taking a homeopathic remedy, avoid consuming tobacco, food or beverages, especially mint of any kind (including that in toothpaste), and caffeine-containing beverages, including coffee, tea, soda, and chocolate. These substances will interfere with the effectiveness of homeopathic remedies. Also, do not handle homeopathics in pill form. Instead, transfer them from their container onto a spoon or other container, then into your mouth.

HOW OFTEN ARE HOMEOPATHIC REMEDIES TAKEN?

When symptoms are acute, remedies may be taken as often as hourly for a short period of time. For chronic problems, remedies may be taken in the morning and at night for longer periods of time.

HOW CAN HOMEOPATHY BENEFIT A WOMAN DURING MENOPAUSE?

While homeopathic remedies can be self-selected at natural foods markets, the guidance of a trained professional may be needed. There are numerous combination formulas which may be useful during menopause and are named for the general conditions they remedy, such as constipation, insomnia and anxiety, menopause, nervousness, restlessness, rheumatism and muscle fatigue, etc. The following single remedies may be useful for specific conditions:

- Aconitum Napellus for restlessness and sleeplessness
- Arum Metallicum for depression
- Belladonna for excitability, restlessness, night sweats and hot

flashes, insomnia, and headache; also for painfully dry and extremely sensitive vagina

- Bellis Perennis for chronic tiredness
- Bryonia for PMS or breast tenderness
- Calcarea Carbonica for chills, muscular weakness and fatigue
- Chamomilla for irritability, hypersensitivity to pain, and insomnia
- Ferrum Metallicum for hot flashes and exhaustion
- Gelsemium Sempervirens for exhaustion and apprehension
- Ignatia Amara for nervousness and emotional stress
- Lac Cuninum for painful, swelling breasts
- Lachesis Mutus for irritability and hot flashes, profuse menstruation or "flooding," thick blood flow, bloating, and irritability
- Lycopodium for dry skin and vagina
- Magnesia Phosphorica for headaches
- Nox Vomica for impatience, irritability and anger, night sweats
- Natrum Muriaticum for irregular periods, "flooding," headache, exhaustion, water retention
- Passiflora Incarnata to calm and soothe the nerves, relieve insomnia
- Pilocarpus Microphyllus for night sweats
- Populus Tremuloides for night sweats
- Pulsatilla for moodiness, sadness, insomnia, joint pain, PMS, hot flashes, and impending involuntary urination
- Salvia for night sweats
- Sanguinaria for hot flashes of the face, hands, and feet
- Sepia for hot flashes, vaginal dryness, thinning hair, constipation, depression, disinterest in sex, irritability, headache, and menstrual "flooding"
- Stramonium for irritability, fearfulness, and anger
- Sulfur for dry itchy skin or vulva, night sweats, and thirst
- Valeriana eases hot flashes and sweating
- Viburnum Opulus for restless sleep and excitability
- Zincum Metallicum for dribble and leak involuntary urination

NATUROPATHY

WHAT IS NATUROPATHY?

Naturopathy is a natural healing approach that focuses strongly on dietary adjustments, eliminating toxic and harmful habits, and by utilizing natural remedies and nutritional supplements.

HOW CAN NATUROPATHY BENEFIT WOMEN DURING MENOPAUSE?

Naturopathy has been shown to be effective in relieving the discomforts many women experience during menopause. The gradual rebalancing and rebuilding of a woman's body can also help to reduce her risks of developing serious health problems later in life.

ARE ALTERNATIVE TREATMENTS COVERED BY HEALTH INSURANCE AND MEDICARE?

Many noninvasive medical treatments are now covered by health insurance and Medicare in the U.S. Although it differs from carrier to carrier and state to state, generally acupuncture, chiropractic care, homeopathy, naturopathy, psychotherapy, and stress reduction training programs such as biofeedback (discussed in the next chapter) are covered. Although insurance will pay for prescription drugs, only some carriers pay for natural remedies and none will pay for vitamin/mineral supplements or herbs.

CHAPTER 6

▲ ▲ ▲

What Lifestyle Changes Can Enhance a Woman's Health With or Without HRT?

The importance of dietary and lifestyle changes is being emphasized today by the U.S. medical community to enhance a woman's overall health and well-being whether or not she takes *HRT* during menopause and into her later years.

Lifestyle changes may help you decide whether you need *HRT* or they may improve the effectiveness of the *HRT* you choose. All doctors will agree that *HRT* alone, without adequate nutritional intake and a routine exercise program, cannot prevent serious health problems that a woman can develop later in life. Studies indicate that women who take *HRT* tend to take better care of their overall health.

IS THERE A BASIC HEALTH AND FITNESS PROGRAM THAT CAN MAKE THE MENOPAUSAL TRANSITION EASIER?

There are general guidelines that all medical experts agree will make your menopausal transition easier whether or not you are taking *HRT*. An overall health and fitness program can be surprisingly effective at encouraging a woman's feelings of physical comfort and emotional well-being during menopause:

- Drink lots of fresh, toxin-free water.
- Adjust your diet and nutritional intake, eliminating foods detrimental to your health and increasing health-affirming foods.

- Take nutritional supplements and/or herbs when needed, based on your individual health profile and your nutritional food intake.

- Undertake a routine, moderate exercise program of at least 30 minutes every day or 60 minutes every other day.

- Learn to reduce stress in your life.

- Develop effective ways to deal with the stress you can't eliminate.

- Avoid self-imposed toxic exposure and environmental toxins. Stop smoking, excessive drinking, and avoid exposure to heavy metals, chemicals, and pesticides.

- Seek professional healthcare support and assistance when you need it.

WHY IS DRINKING PLENTY OF FRESH WATER GOOD FOR A WOMAN'S BODY?

Water may be the most overlooked antidote to aging. Our bodies—at least 75 percent water—require constant replenishment of this essential fluid. Every cell of the body needs water for hydrating skin, regulating body temperature, lubrication, flushing waste and toxins, and transporting nutrients so the body can maintain its balance and support all its functions. Adequate water intake helps your skin stay smooth and prevents tiny wrinkles from forming. Because water flushes the bladder, it often reduces the likelihood of urinary tract infections. Water intake should be increased during hot weather in order to rehydrate your body, even if you do not feel thirsty.

HOW MUCH WATER DOES A WOMAN NEED TO DRINK EVERY DAY?

It has been recommended that you need to drink at least 6 to 8 glasses of clean, pure water every day to maintain optimal health.

IS TAP WATER GOOD ENOUGH?

Tap water is generally not considered beneficial for optimal health, although tap water quality varies from city to city. Most city water is processed and treated in order to remove harmful elements, however, many viruses and bacteria usually remain and in the process chlorine and fluoride are added, which some experts believe are harmful to health and may contribute to bone loss associated with osteoporosis.

WHAT KIND OF WATER IS BEST TO DRINK?

Bottled water is better.

Distilled water, the purest, is widely advocated for use during healing programs. However, continuous use of distilled water over long periods of time may deplete the body of minerals and requires supplementary mineral intake to resupply the body. Purified water is similar to distilled water.

Natural mineral waters contain minerals that are beneficial to the body and must come from a protected underground source. Spring water comes from an underground source that could flow naturally to the surface, but is usually pumped into containers. Artesian water comes from natural wells in rock formations and is pumped out so that it does not come in contact with possible toxins in the soil while being bottled. Natural sparkling water contains natural carbonation and is a good replacement for carbonated sodas.

Sparkling water has CO^2 added to make it fizzy. Club soda is tap water with CO^2 added for fizz and mineral salts added for flavor. Seltzer is tap water with CO^2 added for fizz, but is usually salt-free because no mineral salts are added. Flavored waters may either come from a natural source or from tap water and could have either natural or artificial flavors, as well as sugar or sweeteners.

WHAT DIETARY AND NUTRITIONAL ADJUSTMENTS ARE USUALLY RECOMMENDED FOR A WOMAN DURING AND AFTER MENOPAUSE?

It is important to eliminate foods and beverages that are detrimental to your health and to add foods and beverages that are beneficial to your body by enhancing your vitality, recuperative abilities, and providing nutritional support during this time of dramatic physical changes.

WHAT BEVERAGES ARE DETRIMENTAL TO THE BODY?

Coffee, strong black tea, and sodas are generally considered harmful to the body, except in moderation. Although alcohol consumption is debated, there is no question that excessive alcohol is detrimental. Some healthcare providers believe a glass or two of wine or a beer daily is beneficial to health, but that depends on the individual and her personal and family health profiles.

WHY ARE COFFEE, BLACK TEA, AND SODAS BAD FOR THE BODY?

Most processed sodas, cola drinks, and sweetened carbonated beverages not only contain large amounts of sugar or artificial sweeteners, which are known to be bad for the body, but they also contain phosphorus, which leaches calcium from the bones. This is a particular concern for women during and after menopause when bone loss can accelerate due to lower levels of hormone production.

Coffee, black tea, and some sodas contain large amounts of caffeine and although caffeine in various forms has been used throughout history as a beneficial stimulant, it is the form and quantity in which it is taken into the body that is important.

HOW DOES CAFFEINE BENEFIT THE BODY?

Caffeine naturally provides energy, raises body temperature, suppresses appetite, and increases metabolism.

WHEN IS CAFFEINE BAD?

With excessive consumption, caffeine can be an addictive stimulant. It can raise blood pressure, cause heart palpitations, anxiety and nervousness, digestive and stomach problems, headaches, and sleep disturbance. It can leach vitamins and minerals from the body, contributing to hormonal imbalances and osteoporosis. Caffeine has been linked to breast and uterine fibroid tumors and PMS, heart disease, and high cholesterol.

Your accumulated caffeine consumption may be higher than you think when you consider the numerous sources of caffeine in everyday use in the U.S. Both coffee and tea have large amounts of caffeine. Smaller quantities of caffeine can have a cumulative effect on the body when you consume certain soft drinks, some pain medications, and chocolate, which contains a caffeine-like substance.

Be careful if you decide to eliminate caffeine totally from your diet because you may experience withdrawal symptoms such as severe headaches that can last for several days. Gradually reducing caffeine consumption would probably be in the best health interest of all women.

WHAT DIETARY ADJUSTMENTS ARE GOOD FOR A WOMAN'S BODY DURING AND AFTER MENOPAUSE?

Foods detrimental to your health include refined flours and processed foods, animal fats, and sugar. Your health will benefit if you eat more fresh, whole, natural foods, including grains, nuts, seeds, vegetables, fruits, fish, and poultry.

WHY ARE REFINED FLOURS AND PROCESSED FOODS DETRIMENTAL TO A WOMAN'S HEALTH?

Food in its natural, fresh form is filled with nutrients that are lost when it is refined and processed.

The most significant amounts of vitamins and minerals in grains are in the germ and bran and these are usually removed during the milling process that produces flour. It has been estimated that 30 percent of the average diet consists of grains, usually as refined flour. That is a substantial loss of potential vitamin and mineral consumption in the diet, especially during the middle and later years when a woman's body needs extra nutritional support.

Processed food has usually been exposed to high temperatures, radiation, or chemicals and may need to be reformed to give it texture and artificial colors, and flavors, and preservatives may be added to make it look good, taste good, and last a long time on the supermarket shelf. At this point, if it has any nutritional value, it's most likely because vitamins and minerals have been put back in unnaturally. The end product is food that may look, feel, and taste real, but it's been manufactured. It may supply nutrients to your body, but not in the natural balance foods have in their original form. Further, any chemicals used in food processing and preserving, flavoring, and coloring are foreign substances to your body.

WHY IS IT BETTER FOR A WOMAN TO EAT FRESH FOODS?

A well-balanced diet of fresh foods is more likely to furnish your body with all the elements it needs in order to stay healthy during the menopausal transition and later.

Protein strengthens your body and enhances healing. Complex carbohydrates provide energy and stamina. Soluble fiber helps your body discard waste and toxins, assisting in weight management. Vitamins and minerals are the essential elements for your body to energize and renew itself by stimulating the body's metabolism and helping it convert protein and carbohydrates to tissue and energy.

WHICH VITAMINS AND MINERALS CAN BE BENEFICIAL DURING MENOPAUSE AND WHICH FOODS CONTAIN THEM?

The advice of a healthcare professional with training in nutrition can help you tailor your nutritional intake and supplemental vitamin/mineral dosages to your individual health needs. However, these vitamins, minerals, and other supplements have been found to benefit women during their middle and later years:

- Vitamin A is found in apricots, broccoli, cantaloupe, carrots, lettuce, parsley, spinach, turnips, fish, and dairy products. It is good for the mucous membranes, reproductive system, skin, and eyes and is required for cell regeneration, regulating hormone synthesis and cartilage formation, and supports liver and adrenal gland functions. It is an anti-oxidant that helps protect the body when stressed and resists infection.

Do not take vitamin A supplements if you are taking birth control pills or HRT. Women taking these medications usually have increased levels of vitamin A and do not need to supplement. Vitamin A is also unnecessary if you are taking cod liver oil or fish oil supplements, as they contain high levels of the vitamin, and if you are taking the drug Accutane (isotretinoin), which is made from vitamin A, for a skin condition.

Vitamin B complex (20 different vitamins are included) is found in almonds, brewer's yeast, salmon and other fish, meat and liver, wheat germ, and is essential for almost every function of the body.

Additional intake of these B vitamins may be needed by some women:

- B-5 (calcium pantothenate, pantothenic acid) is found in brewer's yeast, green vegetables, eggs, meat, nuts, wheat germ and bran, whole grains. It reduces stress and aids adrenal function (estrogen production shifts from the ovaries to the adrenals at menopause).

- B-6 (pyridoxine) is found in blackstrap molasses, brewer's yeast, cantaloupe, cabbage, eggs, fish, meat, milk, peanuts, soybeans, walnuts, wheat bran, wheat germ. It has a progesterone effect in the body and decreases water retention and menopause symptoms. More is needed if you are taking estrogen.

• Vitamin C is found in broccoli, brussels sprouts, cauliflower, citrus fruits, green leafy vegetables, parsley, peppers, potatoes, strawberries. It is important for regeneration of body cells, is beneficial to your cardiovascular system, and can alleviate hot flashes.

• Vitamin D is naturally manufactured by your body when it is exposed to sunlight and is also found in fish, fish oils, milk, and dairy products. It is important for healthy bones.

• Vitamin E is found in bee pollen, cold-pressed oils, eggs, green vegetables, peanuts, soybeans, wheat germ, whole grains. It benefits your reproductive organs, cardiovascular system, nerves, and muscles of the skin, and can reduce genital disorders such as vaginal dryness and itching. Vitamin E, along with B-complex, relieves hot flashes and other discomforts associated with menopause including emotional symptoms.

Precaution: a woman with rheumatic heart disease needs to limit her supplemental vitamin E intake.

While taking *HRT*, vitamin E with selenium is recommended. However vitamin E stimulates estrogen in your body, therefore it needs to be taken several hours before or after *HRT*. Taking vitamin E may enhance the effectiveness of *HRT* and you may need to work with your doctor to reduce your estrogen dosage.

Vitamin E can also relieve vaginal dryness. Puncture a capsule and insert a few drops of vitamin E into your vagina.

• Vitamin F (essential fatty acids) is found in virgin cold-pressed oils such as canola, corn, linseed, peanut, safflower, sesame, sunflower, and walnut, as well as in avocados, almonds, peanuts, pecans, sunflower seeds, and walnuts. Essential fatty acids (EFAs) are important for estrogen production and act as a sedative, a diuretic, and aid in alleviating hot flashes. EFAs are essential for cell regeneration and are an anti-toxin, benefiting the circulation, liver, nerves, and skin. EFAs are contained in supplements of evening primrose oil, black currant oil, and flaxseed oil.

Minerals:

- Calcium is found in almonds, green vegetables, dairy products, and sesame seeds. It can alleviate hot flashes when used with vitamin C. Because calcium benefits the nervous system, it can help alleviate emotional symptoms of menopause, such as anxiety and depression, and it contributes to better sleep and relaxation. Calcium and magnesium are essential for bone health, with added boron.

- Iron is found in apricots, eggs, molasses, parsley, red beets, spinach, and whole grains. It is an essential element of healthy blood and necessary to avoid anemia, especially when a woman experiences profuse menstrual bleeding.

- Copper is found in fresh fruits and green vegetables. It is necessary for iron to be absorbed by your body.

- Magnesium is found in eggs, lemons, milk, nuts, sea salt, milk, soy products, and whole grains. It is essential for your body to absorb calcium. It has an anti-aging effect by supporting cell regeneration, relieves hot flashes, and calms nerves.

- Selenium is a trace mineral and antioxidant taken daily in amounts ranging from 50-200 mcg. Studies have shown a connection between selenium deficiency and the pain and swelling of arthritis. Studies also indicate selenium deficiency in breast cancer patients.

- Acidophilus enables the intestines to absorb nutrients by supporting and maintaining your body's production of beneficial bacteria. It can be eaten in cultured food, such as yogurt, kefir, and some milks. Supplements are available at health food stores. Acidophilus capsules can be inserted into your vagina at night to help prevent or alleviate vagina infections.

- Digestive enzymes, including HCl (hydrochloric acid) are essential for the body to assimilate nutrients. Although they are contained in all unprocessed, uncooked foods, it may be necessary to supplement your diet, especially with HCl. Many combination vitamin/mineral formulations contain HCl.

WHAT VITAMINS CAN MAKE HRT MORE EFFECTIVE?

Certain vitamins have been found to have an estrogenic effect in the body and will make *HRT* more effective and possibly necessitate reducing your dosage: vitamins E, B-6, B-12, PABA, folic acid, and pantothenic acid. If you are taking these vitamins or wish to, tell your doctor and discuss your *HRT* dosage adjustment options.

ARE ANY OTHER FOODS ESPECIALLY BENEFICIAL DURING MENOPAUSE?

Some foods have an estrogenic effect in a woman's body and may alleviate the discomforts of menopause without taking *HRT* or they may enhance the effect of *HRT*: soybeans (which contain phytoestrogens), soy foods like tofu, miso, koridofu, aburage, and atuage are generously eaten in Japan, where women rarely have menopausal symptoms. Other foods that have an estrogenic effect in the body and have been shown to be beneficial for relieving the discomforts of menopause are alfalfa, almonds, apples, cashew nuts, corn, cucumbers, oats, peanuts, peas, and wheat.

CAN A WOMAN GET ENOUGH VITAMINS AND MINERALS FROM FOOD OR ARE SUPPLEMENTS NECESSARY?

Most women cannot get enough vital nutrients from today's food because it is grown in nutrient-depleted soil and is exposed to toxins from ground water contamination, pesticides, and chemical fertilizers. Further, processed and junk food diets not only do not provide nutrients to your body, they also deplete the body of stored nutrients.

CAN A WOMAN RELY ON SUPPLEMENTS FOR NUTRITIONAL BALANCE INSTEAD OF BEING CONCERNED ABOUT HER DIET?

Although supplements can be beneficial, they do not contain the complex nutrient balance of fresh wholesome food. Supplements are not as easily assimilated by the body as the nutrients in fresh, wholesome food. At safe levels of intake, supplements are not stored by the body for use when they are needed, but are excreted in the urine. Lower doses of supplements taken along with a nutritious diet are most effective for good health.

Nutritional supplements combined with a healthy diet have been shown to offset the risks of heart attack and osteoporosis for women in later life. See the chapters on *HRT* and your bones and *HRT* and your cardiovascular system.

HOW DOES EXERCISE BENEFIT A WOMAN DURING MENOPAUSE?

Exercise has an anti-aging effect. It strengthens muscles and bones, benefits the cardiovascular system, lowers cholesterol levels, helps regulate weight, increases energy, reduces stress, and improves mental attitude.

WHAT IS THE BEST WAY FOR A WOMAN TO EXERCISE DURING AND AFTER MENOPAUSE?

Regular, moderate weight-bearing exercise is best. Walking at a quick pace for half an hour every day, or one hour every other day of the week is the most widely recommended form of exercise. Yoga is an excellent form of exercise which tones and stretches muscles as it provides aerobic effects. Tennis and stair climbing are also good. Aerobic exercise routines such as bicycling and swimming are good, but need to be combined with appropriate weight-bearing exercise to be beneficial for your bones.

Excessive aerobic exercise that lowers body fat to abnormal levels is detrimental to the hormonal balance of a woman's body.

If you have any symptoms of heart disease, consult a physician before you begin any exercise routine other than walking.

WHY IS STRESS HARMFUL TO A WOMAN DURING AND AFTER MENOPAUSE?

Not all stress is bad. Stress can motivate us, challenge us, and inspire us. And we know that our bodies need to be stressed and stimulated in order to remain strong and healthy.

But stress begins to affect us negatively when our minds tell our bodies we cannot handle it. Our muscles and organs tense up, our breathing becomes shallow, our blood flow is altered, then the mind sends signals to the rest of the body that something is out of balance.

When we are in balance, our glands secrete hormones that regenerate and renew the body. But when we are feeling stressed, our glands are overstimulated, releasing extra hormones in an attempt to regain balance within the body. In turn, the body needs more nutritional support and too quickly utilizes the available nutrients. If adequate nutrients are not made available to the body through our food intake and supplements, the body will draw the nutrients it needs from the body's warehouses, especially from the bones.

All of this can lead to additional hormonal imbalances causing more discomfort during menopause; vitamin, mineral and nutritional deficiencies within the body; and an extra load on the whole body, especially the glands, cardiovascular system, and the bones.

HOW CAN A WOMAN REDUCE THE HARMFUL EFFECTS OF STRESS?

A feeling of well-being is important for women during menopause when they are experiencing more physical changes than at any time during their life since puberty. A positive outlook is very important. Women who take time for daily grooming feel better about themselves and are generally happier and more relaxed about life.

Some doctors prescribe tranquilizers for women who are over-wrought during menopause. But there are numerous non-drug therapies that can help to relieve stress, as well as techniques you can learn to increase relaxation.

WHAT ARE THE NON-DRUG THERAPIES FOR STRESS REDUCTION AND RELAXATION?

Besides dietary changes, vitamins, minerals, herbs, and exercise routines discussed earlier in this chapter, these are some ways you can reduce or better manage stress:

- Acupressure can be self-applied to some parts of your body to reduce tension, as well as to relieve menopausal discomforts.

- Biofeedback is a stress-reduction and relaxation technique that is widely used both by conventional and alternative medical communities. An electronic machine is connected to sensors applied to your skin. The sensors measure your skin temperature and electrical responses as a visual display shows you the effect tension and anxiety has on your body. Once you learn to recognize tension, you are taught techniques to reduce these responses, thus controlling stress effects on your body. Biofeedback is an effective relaxation technique that can help you overcome anxiety, headaches, and insomnia.

- Dance therapy can help you express your emotions while releasing tension in your body and mind. The therapeutic effects of music enhances the activity.

- Deep breathing. When you become aware of your body or mind becoming tense, taking several long, deep breaths will help you relax. Each time as you breathe out, focus on the feeling of your muscles becoming looser and softer.

- Hypnotherapy is a partnership treatment between a patient and doctor that allows the doctor to induce a state of suspended brain function to the region of the brain linked to anxiety, blood pressure, and emotions. While in the suspended state, you can be taught to change the way your brain responds to everyday situations. Studies have shown it helps people feel more relaxed, stop smoking, lose weight, feel less pain, and heal faster.

- Massage relaxes the body by releasing stress in the muscles. Massage is especially effective because it is a period of time to totally surrender your body and energy to a massage therapist who does all the work for you. It can also be effective in helping your body correct imbalances that lead to menopausal discomforts.

- Meditation and prayer can calm the mind, the body, and enhance healing.

- Reflexology can be performed by a massage therapist, reflexologist, or yourself by pressing points on the feet or hands. It relaxes, releases stress, and can adjust imbalances in the body during menopause.

- Visualization and guided imagery are based on the theory that the mind controls the body. You can learn to visualize changes in your body from an unhealthy state to a healthy condition. The technique has been used throughout the history of medicine to quiet the mind and reduce stress, and is believed to lead to faster healing. Studies have shown that guided imagery (visualization) is being used successfully by some cancer patients to shrink their tumors and by people with persistent infections because it appears to boost the body's immune activity. It is also used widely by athletes to improve their performance.

- Yoga, meaning "union" in Sanskrit, assists in integrating the body, emotions, mind, and spirit. Although there are several types of yoga, the variety most commonly and easily practiced in the West is Hatha Yoga. As you stretch and tone the muscles in slow, relaxed positions, the effects of gravity are counteracted, improving your posture, balance, and giving you a feeling of well-being. Because many of the positions increase circulation, yoga can have an aerobic effect as well. Deep breathing and meditation often accompany yoga, enhancing your sense of self and giving you an opportunity to look inward and feel at peace.

CHAPTER 7

The Discomforts of Menopause— What Can You Do About Them?

The effects of menopause on a woman's body are generally divided into two categories. The discomforts women commonly experience during menopause will be addressed in this chapter, including some ways a woman can relieve them with *HRT* or without taking it.

How *HRT* affects the serious physical problems and health risks a woman may develop during menopause or later in life as a result of her hormonal changes will be addressed in subsequent chapters.

WHAT ARE THE MOST COMMON DISCOMFORTS ASSOCIATED WITH MENOPAUSE?

The most common complaints of women during menopause include:

- hot flashes, often accompanied by heart palpitations and night sweats that cause sleep disturbances
- lack of energy
- vaginal dryness
- loss of sexual desire
- body aches and pains.

Some women also experience emotional changes, anxiety, nervousness, or feelings of instability.

WHAT CAN A WOMAN DO TO ALLEVIATE THE DISCOMFORTS OF MENOPAUSE?

HRT often alleviates the discomforts most women experience during menopause. There are also many simple techniques and non-drug therapies a woman can use to reduce the discomforts of menopause. These can be particularly helpful for a woman who cannot take *HRT* or chooses not to take it, or when used in conjunction with *HRT* to lower her dosage requirements.

HOT FLASHES

WHAT IS A HOT FLASH?

A hot flash is a sudden rush of hot energy, usually starting around the breasts and spreading upward to the neck, face, and head. It may be accompanied by sweating, heart palpitations, and a cold damp feeling on the skin.

One supportive husband was overheard saying to his wife, "It's not a hot flash, it's a power surge."

DO ALL WOMEN HAVE HOT FLASHES?

At least 10 percent of menopausal women never have hot flashes; 80 percent have them from time to time but do not find them disturbing; and 10 percent report they are extremely uncomfortable.

WHAT CAUSES HOT FLASHES?

Hot flashes are related to the erratic production of hormones by the ovaries. Although no one knows for sure what causes hot flashes, it is believed they are related to the complex interaction between the ovaries and the brain. It probably involves the pituitary gland as it attempts to stimulate the ovaries into producing hormones, the hypothalamus, the part of the brain that controls body temperature, and the adrenal glands attempting to kick in and take over production of estrogen when the ovaries begin to stop.

The body becomes hotter inside and blood flow to the skin increases in an effort to cool it down. As a result, the skin temperature rises and the heart rate increases. The skin may become red and sweating may occur. As the perspiration evaporates the skin becomes cold, pale, and damp feeling. In a small percentage of women the effects are severe.

HOW LONG DOES A HOT FLASH LAST?

Although every woman is different, the most common length of a hot flash is about 5 minutes. Some have been reported to last as long as half an hour. Usually, a woman senses when it is going to happen. This preflush period lasts for 1 to 4 minutes before the hot flash actually begins. Then the sudden hot feeling occurs and a wave of heat spreads upward from the chest through the body.

DO OTHER DISCOMFORTS COMMONLY ACCOMPANY HOT FLASHES?

Some women experience dizziness or headaches with hot flashes. Other women report that hot flashes are extremely uncomfortable, with accompanying profuse sweating and frightening heart palpitations, however these are rare. Most women are hardly bothered by hot flashes, even when they are aware that they are happening.

DO HOT FLASHES OCCUR DURING ALL THE YEARS OF THE MENOPAUSAL TRANSITION?

Most women who experience hot flashes say they occur for one or two years. About 30 percent have them for five years or longer.

Because hot flashes are related to erratic hormone production by the ovaries, which can last for several years, the patterns of frequency and duration of hot flashes often change in a woman. She may have them for a short period of time and never have them again, she may have them on and off for longer periods of time, or they may stop for a while and recur.

WHEN DO HOT FLASHES USUALLY OCCUR?

Although hot flashes are usually unpredictable, they often occur during the night. When they occur during the day it can be as a result of these circumstances:

- a sudden fright caused by a loud noise or unexpected sound
- situations that are emotionally stressful
- drinking hot liquids or eating hot or spicy foods
- consumption of alcoholic beverages.

WHAT IS THE MOST DISTURBING ASPECT OF HOT FLASHES?

Although hot flashes can be embarrassing when they are severe and occur in public, this is rare.

Probably the most disturbing aspect of hot flashes is that they frequently occur at night and wake a woman from her sleep. The sweating can also make sleepwear and bedding wet. Nighttime hot flashes can have a dramatic impact on a woman during menopause by interrupting her sleep enough to lead to tiredness and lack of energy. This can also contribute to emotional problems associated with sleep deprivation, such as irritability, anxiety, disorientation, nervousness, and even depression.

IS THERE ANYTHING A WOMAN CAN DO TO STOP HOT FLASHES?

HRT usually effectively stops hot flashes. In addition to *HRT*, or while not taking it, there are nutritional and alternative medical therapies that also help alleviate hot flashes. They include:

- dietary changes
- nutritional supplements
- herbs
- homeopathic remedies
- Ayurveda.

WHAT DIETARY CHANGES CAN HELP ALLEVIATE HOT FLASHES?

Besides the overall health-enhancing diet discussed in chapter 6, hot flashes can be alleviated by avoiding large meals, spicy foods, coffee, and by eating a diet rich in phytoestrogens, foods that have an estrogenic effect in the body. In fact, the infrequency of hot flashes experienced by Asian women is associated with their high intake of soy-based foods, which are phytoestrogens. Other foods that may help hot flashes are alfalfa, almonds, apples, carrots, cashew nuts, corn, cucumbers, oats, peanuts, peas, pomegranate seeds, wheat, and yams.

It is also important to drink plenty of fresh, clean water to help regulate your body temperature, especially during warm weather or when your body is overheated from exercise.

WHAT NUTRITIONAL SUPPLEMENTS CAN HELP ALLEVIATE HOT FLASHES?

- Vitamin E at 400 IU twice daily helps regulate estrogen in the body. Add the trace mineral selenium at 100 mcg daily to enhance heart function and help regulate body temperature.

- Vitamin C at 500 to 1,000 mg with each meal supports adrenal gland function, enhances the effectiveness of estrogen, helps regulate body temperature, and strengthens capillaries. A vitamin C supplement with bioflavonoids is even better. It tones blood vessel walls and reduces their dilation during a hot flash.

- B-complex, containing at least 50 mg of each primary B vitamin twice daily, enhances the effectiveness of estrogen in the body.

- Additional vitamin B-5 (pantothenic acid) at 200 to 500 mg daily, supports adrenal gland function.

- Additional PABA (a member of the B vitamin complex) helps keep estrogen levels higher for longer periods of time.

- Bee pollen contains both male and female hormones and can

help relieve hot flashes as well as other discomforts of menopause. Take around 500 mg a day, but discontinue if you develop allergic reaction symptoms, similar to hay fever.

WHICH HERBS CAN HELP ALLEVIATE HOT FLASHES?

Herbs that have been shown to alleviate hot flashes include ginseng, damiana, dong quai, passion flower, and sarsaparilla. Your healthcare professional might also suggest you take other herbs that might be helpful during the menopausal transition, as discussed in chapter 5.

CAN HOMEOPATHY HELP RELIEVE HOT FLASHES?

Homeopathic remedies that can relieve hot flashes are Belladonna, Ferrum Metallicum, Lachesis Mutus, Lechesis, Pulsatilla, Sanguinaria, and Valeriana. Your healthcare professional might also suggest you take other specific homeopathic remedies for discomfort during menopause.

HOW DOES AYURVEDA HELP ELIMINATE HOT FLASHES?

Ayurveda views hot flashes as excess of pitta (the fire element). Women experiencing hot flashes are advised to eliminate or cut down on cayenne, garlic, ginger, onions, and highly acidic foods such as berries, oranges, grapefruits, and tomatoes. It is best to avoid foods that are hot in temperature, as well as hot tubs, very hot baths, saunas, steam baths, and exercise in extreme heat. Drinking alcoholic beverages is believed to aggravate hot flashes in some women.

LACK OF ENERGY

WHAT CAUSES A LACK OF ENERGY DURING MENOPAUSE?

Lack of energy is a common complaint of women during menopause. Generally, as a woman's body changes, it requires additional support and assistance in order to keep it operating efficiently. This support can come from good nutritional intake of foods, supplements, and herbs.

Lack of energy during menopause often is due to inadequate rest and relaxation, which are essential during this time of life. A woman who experiences hot flashes that interrupt her sleep may quickly become fatigued and lack energy.

Extreme lack of energy could also be a result of reduced levels of testosterone in a woman's body. Although the amount of testosterone produced by the ovaries is very small, it definitely has an energizing effect in your body.

Unrelated health problems may also cause fatigue. A complete physical examination may indicate the cause.

HOW CAN A WOMAN ENHANCE HER ENERGY DURING MENOPAUSE?

Hormone replacement therapy can increase energy in a woman during menopause and has been shown to reduce the emotional instability that sometimes accompanies menopause and can cause excessive fatigue. *HRT* that includes testosterone may be suggested by your physician in cases of extreme fatigue.

Dietary changes, supplemental intake of specific nutrients, exercise, and relaxation techniques can be surprisingly effective ways to enhance energy during menopause, as discussed in chapter 6.

WHAT NUTRITIONAL SUPPLEMENTS ENHANCE ENERGY?

- Calcium (1000 mg) and magnesium (500 mg) at bedtime can help a woman get a good night's sleep, to awaken with more energy the next day.
- If your doctor determines that inadequate thyroid function (discussed in chapter 8) is a problem, the iodine in sea vegetables such as kelp can be taken in supplemental form.
- If an iron deficiency exists from excessive menstrual bleeding, supplemental intake of iron can help.

- Inadequate adrenal function can contribute to a lack of energy. If that is the case, supplements for hot flashes discussed earlier in this chapter may be helpful.
- Herbs that have a rejuvenating effect in the body, such as bee pollen, gota kola, or alfalfa can be taken early in the day.

VAGINAL DRYNESS

WHAT CAUSES VAGINAL DRYNESS DURING MENOPAUSE?

Vaginal dryness during menopause is directly related to reduced amounts of hormone production by the body. The vaginal lining contains glands that secrete fluid when stimulated by hormones produced by the ovaries.

WHAT CAN A WOMAN DO TO ALLEVIATE VAGINAL DRYNESS?

Hormone replacement therapy is known to alleviate vaginal dryness. Supplemental use of estrogen or natural progesterone cream inserted in the vagina are also effective.

There are numerous supplements and non-drug treatments that can alleviate vaginal dryness.

WHICH SUPPLEMENTS CAN HELP TO RELIEVE VAGINAL DRYNESS?

The supplements discussed earlier in this chapter which enhance estrogen production for alleviating hot flashes may also reduce vaginal dryness. In addition:

- Vitamin E capsules can be punctured and a few drops inserted into the vagina for lubrication.
- Aloe vera gel can be used as a lubricant.
- K-Y jelly and other over-the-counter remedies such as *Replens,* are effective for relief of vaginal dryness.
- Regular sexual activity, either with a partner or alone, also enhances lubrication of the vagina.

IS VAGINAL DRYNESS A SYMPTOM OF A MORE SERIOUS CONDITION?

Initially, vaginal dryness can be disturbing because it makes sexual intercourse uncomfortable. Vaginal dryness also occurs at the same time tissue in the vagina becomes thinner and more easily damaged or torn. This can result in vaginal bleeding or an increased likelihood of infections.

More serious health conditions such as vaginal atrophy usually develop after the completion of menopause when hormone levels in the body are very low, as discussed in chapter 12.

LOSS OF SEXUAL DESIRE

WHAT CAUSES LOSS OF SEXUAL DESIRE DURING MENOPAUSE?

Loss of sexual desire during menopause does not usually result from loss of hormone production within the body, although lack of testosterone could cause that effect. Testosterone, the androgen manufactured in small amounts by the ovaries, is sometimes linked to sexual desire.

However, vaginal dryness caused by hormonal changes can make sexual intercourse painful and that can douse the flames of sexual desire.

Loss of sexual desire can also be the result of the emotional uncertainty a woman may feel because her image of herself is changing along with her body.

Many women report increased sexual desire after menopause. They say their inability to become pregnant is liberating and they can focus mainly on the emotional and sensory feelings of attraction or love for another person.

DOES A WOMAN'S LEVEL OF SEXUAL EXCITEMENT CHANGE DURING MENOPAUSE?

The hormonal and circulatory changes during menopause can

increase sexual arousal time and the need for more stimulation to reach orgasm.

WHAT CAN A WOMAN DO TO REGAIN LOST SEXUAL DESIRE DURING MENOPAUSE?

Hormone replacement therapy or the alternatives discussed earlier in this chapter to relieve vaginal dryness can usually give a woman a general feeling of well-being that enhances her sexual desire. A woman with severe loss of sexual desire can discuss with her doctor the possibility of having her *HRT* include testosterone.

CAN NON-DRUG THERAPIES RESTORE LOST SEXUAL DESIRE DURING MENOPAUSE?

An overall health-enhancing diet, exercise, and lifestyle can be beneficial to the body, mind, and sexuality of a woman during menopause. Enhancing your self-image is probably the best aphrodisiac you could find.

Although it is said that specific foods are aphrodisiacs, that has not been proven. Still, foods that will increase the vitality needed for sexual energy include: brewer's yeast, broccoli, cantaloupe, carrots, chocolate, cinnamon, eggs, peas, sea foods, soy products, and spinach.

Herbs that have been used as sexual stimulants include:

- Ginseng is considered a powerful aphrodisiac, although it can be too stimulating for some women to take.
- Yohimbe stimulates testosterone, although it can be detrimental to existing heart, liver, or kidney problems.
- Hops has a powerful estrogen effect in the body and it is sometimes recommended that hops tea be taken as a sexual stimulant.
- Parsley tea is said to be a mild sexual stimulant.
- A tea made of savory and fenugreek is an old French remedy for sexual stimulation.

EMOTIONAL CHANGES

WHAT CAUSES EMOTIONAL CHANGES IN A WOMAN DURING MENOPAUSE?

The reduced production of estrogen and progesterone by the ovaries have an effect on your nervous system and can contribute to emotional changes during menopause in other ways, too. Progesterone in particular is linked to PMS, and is widely used in England for its treatment. Dramatically increased levels of progesterone beginning during the second trimester of pregnancy are said to account for the feeling of euphoria many pregnant women experience.

A change in the menstrual cycles definitely affects a woman's emotions because her body feels and acts different than before menopause.

The other discomforts of menopause, such as hot flashes, heart palpitations, and night sweats can make it difficult for a woman to get adequate rest. This unquestionably leads to feelings of forgetfulness, anxiety, nervousness, and in severe cases, depression.

ARE SOME EMOTIONAL CHANGES DURING MENOPAUSE STRICTLY PSYCHOLOGICAL?

Usually, the emotional changes that occur during menopause are related to a woman's physical changes, but are not caused by them. The physical changes that occur in almost every part of a woman's body during menopause sometimes make her feel as though her body belongs to someone else and it may take time to get used to these changes.

A woman may begin to feel and see herself starting to age. She may begin to view her body and her sexuality differently as she needs to make changes in her sex life because of vaginal changes.

Sometimes emotional changes during menopause are not related to physical changes, but are caused by the lifestyle or environmental factors of everyday life. The pressures many women experience during the middle years of life can be difficult to handle emotionally. Stress reduction techniques discussed in chapter 6 may be helpful when that is the case.

HOW ARE EMOTIONAL PROBLEMS TREATED DURING MENOPAUSE?

Emotional changes directly related to diminished hormone production can often be alleviated by *HRT.* However, some studies have shown that taking estrogen can cause a woman to experience more depressive symptoms.

Some doctors prescribe tranquilizers or antidepressants for a woman who has severe emotional problems during menopause. There are also numerous natural methods for balancing the emotions and relieving anxiety, as discussed in chapters 5 and 6, that do not have the side effects of tranquilizers and antidepressants.

Emotional changes alone are usually not a good reason to take *HRT.*

WHAT NATURAL METHODS ARE USEFUL FOR EMOTIONAL CHANGES DURING MENOPAUSE?

Dietary changes and exercise are effective for relieving emotional problems during menopause. Eliminating stimulating foods or depressants such as sugar, coffee, chocolate, alcohol, and cigarettes has been shown to calm the nerves and balance the emotions.

Supplemental intake of calcium, magnesium, and B-complex vitamins has a calming effect in the body. Herb teas are effective, including those containing camomile, passion flower, hops, catnip, skullcap, and peppermint.

Aromatherapy can be extremely calming to the nerves and emotions. Sage eases tension and balances hormones. Camomile and lavender enhance relaxation and calm nerves. Thyme can alleviate insomnia and improve circulation. Use a few drops of basil, cypress, rosemary, and thyme in a nice warm bath.

Homeopathic remedies and Bach flower remedies can be especially helpful for emotional changes during menopause. Also extremely beneficial are massage, reflexology, and relaxation techniques and therapies such as biofeedback, guided imagery, hypnotherapy, yoga, dance therapy, listening to music, meditation, and prayer.

BODY ACHES AND PAINS

WHY DO SOME WOMEN EXPERIENCE BODY ACHES AND PAINS DURING MENOPAUSE?

Body aches and pains, general discomfort in the bones, and backache, are common complaints of women during menopause. It is known that the sudden drop in hormones during and after menopause is a catalyst for bone loss, although osteoporosis itself has no real symptoms. Backache, especially in the lower back, can be caused by energy changes in the pelvic organs.

WHAT CAN A WOMAN DO ABOUT BODY ACHES AND PAIN DURING MENOPAUSE?

HRT may alleviate some of the aches and pains a woman experiences during menopause.

Dietary adjustments can enhance the rejuvenative abilities of the body and make the work of the digestive system easier and more effective.

Massage, acupuncture, and acupressure are especially beneficial for a woman at this time, and homeopathic remedies can provide relief as well.

Exercise is beneficial for the body in every way, as discussed in chapter 6. Women who do not feel up to strenuous activity may select gentle stretching and yoga, which are extremely relaxing. Dance therapy can be either relaxing or invigorating. It can be a woman's way of celebrating life, a ritual performed by people throughout the ages in every culture.

CHAPTER 8
▲ ▲ ▲

What Are the Effects of HRT on Your Appearance?

Taking *HRT* during and after menopause has been shown to affect a woman's body shape, hair, and skin both positively and negatively, depending on the woman and the types and dosages of the hormones she is taking. *HRT* appears to delay the effects of aging for a time, but does not stop the natural aging process, which can be strongly influenced by a woman's genetic factors, as well as her diet and lifestyle.

HOW DOES ESTROGEN AFFECT A WOMAN'S APPEARANCE?

Estrogen has been shown to have a beneficial effect on a woman's skin and breasts by causing them to seem fuller, with less sagging. However, this plumping-up effect that pleases some women causes others to complain that taking estrogen results in fluid retention, a bloated feeling, and weight gain. Some women have experienced hair loss while taking estrogen.

WHAT EFFECTS DO PROGESTINS HAVE ON A WOMAN'S APPEARANCE?

Because progestins affect the uterus, women taking them along with estrogen have complained of abdominal bloating and fluid retention.

DO WOMEN TAKING NATURAL PROGESTERONE HAVE THE SAME COMPLAINTS?

Natural progesterone is identical in molecular structure to the progesterone produced by the body, as compared to molecularly altered progestins. Therefore, natural progesterone does not produce the same negative effects on the body as progestins. It has been reported that natural progesterone reduces fluid retention and has an antiwrinkling effect on the skin.

HOW DOES TAKING TESTOSTERONE AFFECT A WOMAN'S APPEARANCE?

Because testosterone is a masculinizing hormone, taking it can result in unwanted hair growth, weight gain, and muscle mass increase.

BODY SHAPE

WHAT BODY SHAPE CHANGES MIGHT A WOMAN EXPERIENCE WHILE TAKING HRT?

Not all women do experience body shape changes while taking *HRT*, but many women complain of abdominal bloating, fluid retention, and weight gain.

Changes in the breasts are also quite common, including breasts that feel more tender and fuller. Breast changes while taking *HRT* are potentially serious and will be addressed in chapter 10.

DO WOMEN NOT TAKING HRT EXPERIENCE BODY-SHAPE CHANGES DURING AND AFTER MENOPAUSE?

Body-shape changes and redistribution of fat during menopause is not uncommon, with many women experiencing greater fat accumulation in the stomach area and thighs. Although this may seem upsetting as it occurs, it may also be beneficial by plumping up skin that is naturally losing its firmness, especially after menopause. A little extra fat may also help alleviate the discomforts of menopause because the body converts the androgens in fat to estrogen.

Women not taking *HRT* may experience breast changes, as discussed in chapter 10, during and after menopause, as the estrogen production in their bodies diminishes dramatically.

DOES MENOPAUSE ITSELF CAUSE A WOMAN TO GAIN WEIGHT?

It is generally agreed that menopause does not cause weight gain. Any weight gain and fluid retention associated with the menopausal years is usually related to lack of exercise and poor eating habits. However, weight gain or weight loss can also be associated with thyroid gland malfunction.

WHY DOES TAKING HRT CAUSE SOME WOMEN TO GAIN WEIGHT?

While the reasons are not certain, it is believed to be caused by a combination of factors: fluid retention that is known to be associated with taking *HRT,* thyroid gland malfunction, or lifestyle patterns such as poor eating habits and lack of exercise that generally lead to weight gain.

HOW DOES A WOMAN'S THYROID GLAND FUNCTION AFFECT HER WEIGHT?

The thyroid gland, located in the lower throat area, regulates a woman's metabolism. When thyroid function is too low (hypothyroidism) a woman may experience weight gain, lack of energy, dry skin, brittle nails, dull hair, sometimes accompanied by hair thinning, a slow pulse, and intolerance to cold.

When thyroid function is too high (hyperthyroidism) a woman may experience weight loss, feelings of anxiety and nervousness, inability to relax even when tired, a fast pulse, an intolerance to heat, and sometimes heart palpitations.

Thyroid gland malfunction is also believed to cause estrogen imbalances in the body.

HOW DOES A WOMAN KNOW IF HER THYROID GLAND FUNCTION IS NORMAL?

Your physician can conduct various blood tests to evaluate your thyroid function.

If your thyroid function is evaluated, keep in mind that various medications can affect thyroid tests, so be sure to tell your physician if you are taking: *HRT* or birth control pills, aspirin, cough medicine containing iodine, corticosteroids, or dilantin.

WHAT CAUSES THE THYROID GLAND TO MALFUNCTION?

The reasons any glands malfunction in the endocrine system are not easily determined because the function of one gland affects the others. The ovaries are one of the seven primary endocrine glands; the others are the pancreas, adrenals, thymus, thyroid, pituitary, and hypothalamus. Thyroid imbalances seem to occur during perimenopause because the thyroid gland interacts with the pituitary gland as it attempts to stimulate ovulation. Stress seems to have a dramatic effect on thyroid function one way or the other. Diet and nutritional intake may also affect your thyroid gland function.

WHAT CAN A WOMAN DO IF HER THYROID FUNCTION IS ABNORMAL?

Medications are prescribed for cases of extreme thyroid malfunction. However, these must be taken with caution because thyroid medications can increase a woman's risk of osteoporosis, as discussed in chapter 9.

Less extreme thyroid malfunction may be influenced by dietary adjustments and nutritional supplements.

WHAT DIETARY ADJUSTMENTS AND SUPPLEMENTS HELP A WOMAN WITH LOW THYROID ACTIVITY?

Low thyroid function can be caused by lack of iodine, zinc, and copper in the diet. These can be supplied to the body by eating kelp or seaweed, cantaloupe, cod liver oil, fish, beans, chard or turnip greens, peanuts, soy foods, sunflower seeds, or supplements derived from sea vegetables such as kelp and dulse. However, iodine supplements should be taken in extremely limited amounts so as not to throw the thyroid imbalance off to the other extreme. It is best to discuss this issue with a healthcare professional before trying it.

Foods that suppress thyroid function include cabbage, rutabagas, and turnips. Certain drugs and chemicals can also suppress thyroid function, including estrogen (especially the high doses taken in birth control pills), antidiabetic drugs, and sulfa drugs, as well as thyocyanide, a chemical found in cigarette smoke, and fluoride in tap water.

WHICH DIETARY AND SUPPLEMENTAL ADJUSTMENTS HELP A WOMAN WITH HIGH THYROID ACTIVITY?

An overactive thyroid depletes the body of calcium (discussed in chapter 9), essential fatty acids, and vitamins B-1 and B-6 (take a B-complex supplement and extra B-1 and B-6). High thyroid function can also benefit from foods or supplements containing vitamins C, D, and E.

FLUID RETENTION

WHY DOES TAKING HRT CAUSE FLUID RETENTION?

HRT, as well as aspirin and antibiotics, can obstruct the body's utilization of vitamins B-6, B-12, and folic acid, causing fluid retention.

WHAT CAN A WOMAN DO TO ALLEVIATE FLUID RETENTION WHILE TAKING HRT?

Your doctor may suggest a prescription diuretic for fluid retention, however, it is usually not necessary unless serious fluid congestion threatens the health of your heart or lungs. Prescription diuretics can negatively affect blood cholesterol levels and diabetic conditions, as well as deplete the body of magnesium, potassium, sodium, and B vitamins. This can affect your cardiovascular health, as discussed in chapter 11.

Many natural diuretics are very effective and safer for most women to take.

WHAT NATURAL DIURETICS CAN A WOMAN TAKE TO REDUCE FLUID RETENTION?

Drinking plenty of fresh water is the best way to start. Fluid retention is usually caused by not enough water. When your body becomes dehydrated it holds water in an effort to balance itself.

Limit your salt intake, as well as sugars, starches, meats, and dairy products that require more water for the body to dissolve them. Eat foods that have a diuretic effect, including asparagus, celery, cucumbers, kiwi fruit, leafy green vegetables, and parsley.

Vitamin B complex with extra B-6 is an effective diuretic, as is vitamin C.

The herbs cornsilk, dandelion, horsetail, juniper, and uva ursi are effective diuretics, especially in tea form.

SKIN

WHAT HAPPENS TO A WOMAN'S SKIN WHEN HER NATURAL HORMONE LEVELS DECLINE DURING MENOPAUSE?

The skin, as the largest organ of the body, seems to be especially sensitive to the hormonal changes taking place in a woman's body during menopause. The skin has a thin outer layer called the epidermis, and a thick deeper level called the dermis. The dermis, composed mostly of protein collagen and elastin fibers, also contains blood vessels, sensory nerves, and lymph, oil, and sweat glands that nourish hair follicles and the thin outer epidermal layer of skin. Collagen makes your skin thick, toned, and elastic.

Skin cells are constantly renewing themselves in the same

way as all other cells in your body with the help of hormones that assist in breaking down old cells and stimulating the growth of healthy new cells.

As a woman's hormone production decreases, so does the ability of her skin cells to reproduce, resulting in less collagen. In turn the skin becomes thinner, with less fat and muscle to support it, as well as having diminished moisture content. At the same time the deep tissues are contracting, the thin upper layer of skin becomes less elastic and resilient so it starts to sag and wrinkle.

HOW IS ESTROGEN BENEFICIAL FOR A WOMAN'S SKIN?

Estrogen makes the skin feel fuller and more resilient because it encourages skin cells to take up more water. It causes fat to be distributed within the deep skin layers, giving it support and firmness. Estrogen aids collagen protein production within the skin, helping it maintain a healthy thickness.

WILL TAKING ESTROGEN HELP A WOMAN'S SKIN IF SHE ALREADY HAS WRINKLES?

It has been reported that taking estrogen will stop the development of wrinkles to some degree, as well as minimizing existing wrinkling to some extent. However, nothing is known to stop the natural aging process entirely. Because of the potential serious side effects of *HRT*, most doctors will not prescribe *HRT* for a woman who does not otherwise need it, simply because it may delay skin wrinkling for a time.

DO THIN WOMEN USUALLY GET WRINKLED SKIN SOONER THAN HEAVIER WOMEN?

Women with more body fat appear to maintain less wrinkled skin longer than thin women. Heavier women usually have more estrogen stored in body fat, their body fat supports the outer layer of the skin, and they usually have more fluid content in their skin.

HOW LONG DOES IT TAKE FOR THE BENEFICIAL EFFECTS OF HRT TO SHOW UP IN A WOMAN'S SKIN?

If your skin has already started to change because of diminished hormone production in your body and you begin taking estrogen, it will probably take several months before you will see an improvement in your skin.

WHAT CAN A WOMAN DO TO MAINTAIN YOUNGER LOOKING SKIN AFTER MENOPAUSE WITH OR WITHOUT HRT?

Whether or not you choose to take *HRT* for health reasons after menopause, there are some general guidelines you can follow to maintain healthy looking skin:

- Drink at least six to eight glasses of fresh, toxin-free water every day to keep your skin hydrated from the inside. Avoid fluoridated water. Fluoride contributes to skin wrinkling and weakens bones, ligaments, muscles, and tendons, speeding up the aging process.

- Supply moisture to your skin from the outside as well. Use a good moisturizer on your skin at all times and avoid soaps that cause your skin to become dry. A humidifier can help keep your environment moister if you live in a dry climate or if you heat your home during cold months.

- Avoid excessive exposure to skin-damaging sun. Protect your skin with sunscreen during outdoor activity.

- Exercise regularly to improve blood circulation to your skin while toning your muscles.

- Avoid rapid weight loss if you are overweight and want to reduce. A slower weight-loss program will allow your skin to adjust instead of wrinkle, by shrinking along with any fat and fluid supporting it.

- Don't smoke cigarettes.

ARE THERE SPECIAL FOODS OR VITAMINS A WOMAN CAN TAKE TO MAINTAIN HEALTHY SKIN?

The total health diet discussed in chapter 6 featuring fresh, unprocessed foods is a good beginning. Specific vitamins and minerals that have been shown to benefit the skin include:

- The antioxidants, vitamin A and beta-carotene, vitamin E, and the mineral selenium.
- Vitamin C promotes collagen production.
- Vitamin F (essential fatty acids—EFAs) supports the fatty layer of the skin and protects against skin dehydration.

ARE THERE ANY HERBS THAT ARE BENEFICIAL FOR THE SKIN?

Your healthcare professional may suggest you take the herbs discussed in chapter 5 to enhance your overall health and also benefit your skin during menopause. An herb that is especially helpful for skin is horsetail, sometimes called shave grass (equisetum arvense). It contains silica, a component of collagen in the skin, hair, nails, bones, and teeth. It is said that horsetail enhances youthfulness of the body.

DOES PERSPIRING MORE DURING MENOPAUSE DEHYDRATE A WOMAN'S SKIN?

It is important for a woman who perspires more during menopause to rehydrate her body and her skin by drinking plenty of fresh water, eating a nutritious diet of fresh foods, especially those high in magnesium and potassium such as avocados, bananas, barley, brown rice, oats, potatoes, salmon, seeds and nuts, tuna, and turkey.

DOES HRT STOP EXCESSIVE PERSPIRATION?

Androgens, male hormones produced by a woman's adrenal glands and ovaries, stimulate sweat glands in the deep skin layer. Increased

117

perspiration may occur during menopause if enough estrogen is not present to balance the androgens. Often *HRT* can eliminate excessive perspiration some women experience during menopause.

HAIR

DO ALL WOMEN EXPERIENCE CHANGES IN THEIR BODY HAIR DURING MENOPAUSE?

Estrogen stimulates the growth of sexual hair on a woman's body and inhibits the growth of unwanted hair on the face, legs, and arms. During menopause, as estrogen production diminishes, it is not uncommon for a woman to see a decrease in her pubic hair and underarm hair. Sometimes the hair on a woman's head becomes dryer and coarser during menopause.

While estrogen production becomes erratic or diminishes, the body continues to produce androgens, causing an imbalance that may result in growth of unwanted hair on the legs, arms, and sometimes a few coarse hairs grow on a woman's chin or the side of her face.

WHY DO SOME WOMEN EXPERIENCE THINNING HAIR OR LOSS OF HAIR ON THEIR HEADS DURING MENOPAUSE?

The follicles that contain the roots of hairs are located in the deep tissue layer of the skin. During menopause, when estrogen levels drop or become erratic, the tissue surrounding the hair follicles loses collagen and provides less support. Blood flow and energy flow through the nerves, also located in the deep skin layer, may decrease as well, providing less nourishment to the hair follicles.

Stress can cause hair thinning and hair loss by depleting the body of essential B vitamins and causing blood flow to the skin and hair follicles to be diminished.

DOES HRT PREVENT HAIR LOSS AND REVERSE THE HAIR CHANGES WOMEN EXPERIENCE DURING AND AFTER MENOPAUSE?

Some women complain that they experience hair thinning and loss after starting to take *HRT.* This may be because *HRT* can deplete the body of vitamin B-6, a critical nutrient for healthy hair growth.

Generally, *HRT* has been shown to counteract hair loss by resupplying nourishment and support to the hair follicles. It usually prevents unwanted androgen-stimulated hair growth as well.

There is no evidence that hair graying is related to menopause and taking *HRT* is not known to reverse graying hair to its original color.

HOW LONG DOES IT TAKE FOR HRT TO AFFECT A WOMAN'S HAIR?

Once a woman starts taking *HRT,* it will usually take several months before she will see its effects on her hair.

ARE PARTICULAR FOODS AND VITAMINS GOOD FOR A WOMAN'S HAIR?

Adequate nutritional intake helps, as does limiting saturated fats, refined foods, sugars, alcohol, and caffeine. Specific foods that are good for your hair include apples, bananas, carrots, cucumbers, eggs, green peppers, leafy green vegetables, onions, and strawberries. Vitamins and minerals discussed earlier in this chapter that are beneficial for the skin will also benefit the hair, as will the herb horsetail.

WHAT ELSE CAN A WOMAN DO FOR HEALTHIER HAIR DURING AND AFTER MENOPAUSE, WHILE TAKING HRT OR WITHOUT IT?

Practical advice for a woman who wants healthier hair includes:

- Massage your scalp for a few minutes every day to stimulate circulation in the scalp.

- Avoid harsh shampoos and hairstyling products with drying alcohol.
- Use warm water while washing hair and rinse with cool water to increase circulation to the scalp.

CHAPTER 9

▲ ▲ ▲

How Does HRT
Affect Your Bones?

A woman's bones are especially sensitive to the hormonal changes that take place during and after menopause. Hormone replacement therapy is believed to be effective in helping a woman maintain good bone health, especially when combined with adequate nutrition and appropriate lifestyle factors.

WHAT DO HORMONES HAVE TO DO WITH A WOMAN'S BONES?

Bone is living tissue that needs nourishment and stimulation to remain healthy and strong. Hormones stimulate the bones, helping them absorb nutrients, break down aging bone tissue, and build healthy new bone, a process called bone remodeling.

Estrogen stimulates osteoclasts, the cells that break down aging bone cells, dissolve them, and clear a space for new bone to be created. Progesterone stimulates osteoblasts, cells that then come along and form new bone. The process of bone remodeling keeps bones strong and flexible, instead of getting dry and brittle.

Adequate levels of hormones are necessary for the body to continue this process of breaking down aging bone cells and rebuilding new healthy bone. Without hormones, your body cannot properly use calcium, minerals, vitamins, and other nutrients for bone remodeling, and osteoporosis can develop.

WHAT ARE BONES MADE OF?

Bone is made of calcium phosphate crystals connected by collagen protein fibers. That's what makes them strong, yet flexible. Bone is living tissue that needs nourishment and stimulation to remain healthy and serve their various functions within the body.

WHAT ARE THE VARIOUS FUNCTIONS OF BONES WITHIN THE BODY?

Bones create the framework for the body, they protect our organs, they support our muscles, and they are the warehouse where our body stores minerals. Minerals are essential for the proper function of every part of our bodies, but our bodies cannot make minerals. We must get them from our food and supplements.

We have blood and fluids circulating through our bones, just as they do through the rest of our body. The fluids supply nutrients to the bone and at the same time the fluids draw minerals from our bones and carry them to other parts of our body when they are needed.

Our bones stay strong when they can constantly renew their supply of nutrients from the blood and fluid circulating within them.

WHAT IS OSTEOPOROSIS?

Osteoporosis is an excessive deterioration of the bones, leaving them thin and brittle. It develops when the calcium crystals and protein fibers do not get enough nourishment to rebuild and renew themselves to stay strong and flexible.

This can happen because we are not taking in and assimilating enough nutrients or because the bone's nutrient warehouse is being emptied to supply other parts of our bodies. As our body ages, it needs more calcium and minerals.

The effects of osteoporosis usually show up in the later years of life, when bones have deteriorated so much that they easily fracture and break, often causing disability. But because osteoporosis is progressive, it can be avoided or arrested by understanding how the body ages and by taking appropriate action.

DOES TAKING HRT PREVENT OR
REVERSE OSTEOPOROSIS?

Studies have shown that taking *HRT* is beneficial for the bones of most women, especially when combined with adequate nutritional intake and appropriate exercise.

At one time estrogen alone was prescribed for menopausal and postmenopausal women because it alleviated the discomforts of menopause and slowed bone loss. This appeared to result in good bone density, but a woman's bones become more brittle as she gets older because her bone tissue ages as she does.

Knowing that progesterone stimulates the formation of healthy new bone, the medical community began to prescribe progestins along with estrogen. This combination contributed to the formation of new bone to some degree, but did not appear to effectively reproduce natural bone remodeling.

Recent studies indicate that a treatment program of natural progesterone with estrogen, when needed, may be an even more effective treatment for osteoporosis in postmenopausal women. Natural progesterone, which is molecularly identical to the progesterone produced by a woman's ovaries, has been shown to stimulate healthy new bone formation, especially when combined with adequate nutrition and exercise. However, scientific blind studies have not been conducted to confirm the findings of this osteoporosis treatment program that appears to stop progressive osteoporosis and result in the formation of new bone tissue.

IF A WOMAN COMPLETED MENOPAUSE
OVER 3 YEARS AGO, IS IT TOO LATE FOR HER
TO BEGIN TAKING HRT FOR HER BONE HEALTH?

The experts agree that it's never too late to begin *HRT.* However, those who advocate *HRT* consisting of estrogen with progestins will tell you that further bone loss can be avoided, but new bone formation is not realistic.

On the other hand, doctors advocating the use of natural

progesterone with estrogen have seen the formation of healthy new bone in their patients.

The success of either hormone replacement program requires lifestyle adjustments that include adequate nutrition, appropriate weight-bearing exercise, and eliminating destructive lifestyle habits.

HOW LONG DOES A WOMAN NEED TO TAKE HRT TO PREVENT OSTEOPOROSIS?

If you decide to undertake hormone replacement therapy to prevent or treat osteoporosis it is often recommended that it be continued for the rest of your life. Usually, *HRT* is prescribed at the end of menopause because bone loss seems to be most dramatic during the first 3 to 10 years after the ovaries stop producing hormones. After that, the degree of bone loss tapers off dramatically, but continues to decline gradually for the rest of a woman's life.

IF A WOMAN STOPS HRT, WILL THE BENEFITS STAY WITH HER?

The benefits of taking *HRT* usually stop when the treatment does. However, some doctors say even if you do decide to stop taking *HRT* at some point beyond the 3-to-10 year period of greatest bone loss, you're better off because you've maintained more bone mass than you would have otherwise.

HOW CAN A WOMAN KNOW IF SHE NEEDS HRT TO KEEP HER BONES HEALTHY?

There are various ways to assess your overall bone health, including routine medical tests to determine the amount of calcium in your urine or blood, and bone scans that show your bone density. A bone scan measuring your bone density is the best way to determine if you are developing osteoporosis or if you already have significant bone loss.

If you have not had a bone scan before menopause to establish a bone density base line, then your test results will be compared to the average woman. Therefore, women who fall into a high risk category for osteoporosis may choose to have a base line bone scan earlier in life to determine what is normal for them.

WHAT CAUSES OSTEOPOROSIS?

Osteoporosis does not appear to be caused by one particular thing, but by a combination of factors. Worldwide studies have been useful in defining the risk factors of developing osteoporosis, as they are currently understood, based on age and hormone production, heredity, body type, and lifestyle.

WHAT DO A WOMAN'S AGE AND HORMONE PRODUCTION HAVE TO DO WITH OSTEOPOROSIS?

If you are healthy, your bones develop and grow stronger until you are in your thirties. At that point, as your hormone production begins to drop, your bones slowly begin to lose mineral content until menopause begins. After menopause, when your ovaries stop producing hormones, or if your ovaries are surgically removed, comes the period of greatest bone loss, which lasts for 3 to 10 years, depending on your individual health. Then the rate of bone loss slows down, but continues for the rest of your life.

DOES EVERY WOMAN EVENTUALLY DEVELOP OSTEOPOROSIS?

Statistics say that as many as 50 percent of American women are calcium deficient, which can lead to osteoporosis.

Approximately a third of all women show some evidence of osteoporosis by age 60 and 25 percent experience a hip fracture by age 80.

WHAT DO HEREDITY AND BODY TYPE HAVE TO DO WITH OSTEOPOROSIS?

Although no one is certain why, the likelihood of developing osteoporosis appears to be hereditary and more prevalent in women of a certain body type or ethnicity. A woman may need to be more concerned about her bone health if she fits into these higher risk categories:

- A white or Asian female with fair or translucent skin.
- A woman with a history of osteoporosis or hip fracture in her biological family.
- A woman whose body is slender or who has a low muscle mass.

WHY IS HEREDITY A RISK FACTOR FOR DEVELOPING OSTEOPOROSIS?

Studies have shown that osteoporosis probably is hereditary and there are ongoing studies to isolate the gene that causes it. Genetic predisposition to developing osteoporosis may also be related to inherited hormonal patterns in a woman.

WHY ARE THIN WOMEN MORE LIKELY TO DEVELOP OSTEOPOROSIS?

Thin women usually enter menopause earlier than heavier women and heavier women have higher levels of estrogen during and after menopause.

Heavier women stress their bones more in everyday movement because there is more weight pressure on their bones. Also, during and after menopause, as lower levels of hormones are being produced by your ovaries, hormones can be converted from body fat to offset glandular hormonal production decreases.

Perhaps that's why many women develop body fat in the stomach area around the time of menopause. This may be the body's way of creating a natural storehouse of hormones to be used when needed.

DOES THAT MEAN IT'S BETTER TO BE OVERWEIGHT WHEN ENTERING MENOPAUSE?

Being overweight is never beneficial for your overall health.

Maintaining an appropriate, healthy weight for your body type is the best way to stay healthy at any time of life.

ARE THERE SPECIFIC THINGS ALL WOMEN CAN DO TO AVOID OSTEOPOROSIS?

There are basic lifestyle factors that can be controlled in order for a woman to avoid or arrest the development of osteoporosis, including:

- Taking hormone replacement therapy after menopause, if necessary.

- Making dietary changes that provide adequate nutritional support to the body.

- Eliminating destructive dietary choices by avoiding excessive sugar consumption, excessive caffeine consumption by drinking coffee and tea, eating chocolate, excessive regular hard liquor consumption, and excessive consumption of red meat, processed, and refined foods.

- Developing and maintaining an appropriate weight-bearing exercise routine.

- Reducing the destructive effects of stress and anxiety on the body.

- Stop smoking cigarettes.

- Avoid exposure to environmental toxins and heavy metals such as lead, chlorine, and fluoride in drinking water, aluminum in antiperspirants, medications, and cookware.

- Avoid as much as possible the long-term use of thyroid, arthritis, or asthma medications, antibiotics, diuretics, or laxatives.

- Get professional help to overcome eating disorders such as bulimia, anorexia nervosa, or a serious loss of appetite resulting in low caloric intake and malabsorption of nutrients by the body.

HOW DOES WHAT A WOMAN EATS AFFECT HER BONES?

All factors considered, the importance of good food choices cannot be overemphasized as a first step toward healthy bones.

Adequate nutrition from a healthy diet builds bones throughout your life, helps your bones stay strong as you get older, and contributes to the overall good health of your body and mind.

Poor food choices and consumption can block bone building, cause your bones to deteriorate faster, and adversely affect your physical health and emotional well-being.

WHAT FOODS CONTRIBUTE TO GOOD BONE HEALTH?

A well-balanced diet of fresh, unprocessed foods in the form of whole grains, vegetables, and fruits is best. Some studies show that vegetarians who follow a low-fat, non-junk food diet have healthier bones when they enter menopause, and they lose bone at a slower rate after menopause.

Foods that contribute to good bone health include those with plenty of calcium, magnesium, and potassium, such as broccoli, leafy green vegetables, sprouts, carrots, sea vegetables such as kelp, fish and seafood, eggs, yogurt, kefir, bananas, apples, cranberries, apricots, dried fruits, nuts and seeds, beans, soy products such as tofu and miso, and molasses. Also, apple cider vinegar can be used as a salad dressing on fresh vegetables to help the body absorb calcium by raising the pH (alkalinity) of the body.

WHAT DIETARY ADJUSTMENTS CAN BE MADE TO ELIMINATE FOODS THAT ARE DETRIMENTAL TO BONE HEALTH?

- Consume dairy products and salt in moderation.
- Avoid red meats and reduce animal protein and fat consumption.
- Avoid eating refined flours, processed and junk foods.
- As much as possible, eliminate from your diet sugar, caffeine, caffeine-containing foods, and soft drinks.

WHY IS REFINED SUGAR BAD FOR THE BONES?

It is well known that refined sugar is not nutritious and is high in calories. Studies have shown that sugar intake results in a measured increase in calcium excreted in the urine, suggesting that sugar depletes the body of calcium. If over 90 percent of your body's calcium is in the bones, sugar consumption is likely to leach calcium from the bone, thus reducing its calcium content.

A British study found that ingesting sucrose caused an increase in blood cortisol levels in healthy volunteers. The adrenal gland naturally secretes corticosteroid, a cortisonelike hormone, in controlled amounts as needed by the body. Too much corticosteroid can cause osteoporosis by interfering with absorption of calcium and the retention of potassium by the body. This suggests that eating too much sugar may have the same affect on your body, causing your bones to become thinner.

WHY IS CAFFEINE BAD FOR THE BONES?

Studies indicate that caffeine causes calcium to be lost from the body. The higher your caffeine consumption, the greater the calcium loss. Restricting your caffeine consumption is known to benefit your bone health.

IS IT ALL RIGHT TO DRINK DECAFFEINATED COFFEE?

Coffee disturbs the pH balance of your body, making it more acidic. After drinking coffee your body tries to rebalance its own pH by drawing calcium from your bones.

ARE CAFFEINE-FREE SOFT DRINKS BAD FOR THE BONES?

Caffeine-free soft drinks may still be loaded with sugar or artificial sweeteners, which are both bad for the body. But even worse than that, soft drinks are high in phosphorus.

The calcium/phosphorus balance of the body, with twice as much calcium as phosphorus, is very important for good bone health. Excessive phosphorus intake throws off that balance and causes calcium to be excreted in the urine.

WHY ARE REFINED FLOURS AND PROCESSED FOODS BAD FOR THE BONES?

Refined flours and processed foods contain a low nutritional intake for the amount of food that is eaten. Their consumption provides empty calories to a woman's body during and after menopause when nutritional intake is very important for maintaining good bone health.

WHY ARE ANIMAL PROTEIN AND FATS BAD FOR THE BONES?

Meat contains twenty-five times more phosphorus than calcium, therefore excessive meat consumption disturbs the healthy calcium/phosphorus balance of the body (twice as much calcium as phosphorus). Studies have shown that the urinary excretion of calcium increases when animal protein and fats are consumed.

WHY IS A HIGH SODIUM INTAKE BAD FOR THE BONES?

It appears that high sodium intake may result in excess calcium excretion in the urine. Some individuals are hypersensitive to salt and the effect is dramatically magnified with even moderate salt intake.

WHY SHOULD DAIRY INTAKE BE MODERATE? AREN'T DAIRY PRODUCTS A GOOD SOURCE OF CALCIUM?

Dairy products are a good source of calcium, however, they also have drawbacks. The fat content of the most calcium-rich dairy products could be a problem for women who need to be on a low-fat diet. The butterfat in dairy products helps the body absorb calcium and other nutrients, so whole milk or cheese products are a better source of calcium than non-fat or low-fat dairy products. Also, pasteurized milk is sometimes difficult for women to digest as they get older. Some experts claim synthetic vitamin D added to milk can deplete the body of magnesium.

130

Cultured dairy products, especially yogurt with active cultures, may be the best choice for dairy intake because it is more easily digested and the beneficial bacteria promotes absorption of nutrients through the intestines.

IS ICE CREAM A GOOD SOURCE OF CALCIUM?

Yes. However, most ice cream is loaded with sugar, which has no nutritional value, and it is generally agreed that refined sugar is detrimental to the health of most people.

WHAT OTHER FOODS ARE A GOOD SOURCE OF CALCIUM?

Besides dairy products, many other foods are good sources of calcium, including leafy green vegetables, figs and cranberries, salmon, sardines, almonds and sunflower seeds, whole grains, dried beans and soybean foods such as tofu, sprouts, sea vegetables such as kelp and dulse, molasses, and some herbs.

Alfalfa has a very high calcium content and is the food eaten by most dairy cows.

HOW MUCH CALCIUM INTAKE IS NEEDED FOR HEALTHY BONES?

The recommended daily allowance (RDA) of calcium for the average adult is 1000 mg daily. However, it is suggested that women increase their daily intake of calcium to 1500 mg during and after menopause.

IS IT POSSIBLE TO GET ENOUGH CALCIUM FROM FOOD OR ARE SUPPLEMENTS ALWAYS NEEDED?

Calcium derived from a healthy diet is better for two reasons. A calcium-rich diet supplies other nutrients that your body needs as well. A well-balanced diet is necessary for the body to efficiently assimilate and utilize all the nutrients it needs for optimal performance and maintenance.

However, without consistent, conscientious effort, it is usually difficult to get enough calcium and other nutrients from food during and after menopause when the nutritional requirements of your body increase. The dietary calcium intake of the average woman is estimated to be about 400 to 500 mg a day. Therefore, a daily calcium supplement of 500 to 1000 mg is suggested for most women over 35.

WHAT OTHER MINERALS AND VITAMINS ARE IMPORTANT FOR BONE HEALTH?

Various minerals and vitamins interact within the body for proper metabolism and assimilation of all the nutrients you ingest, but these particular nutrients are important for good bone health:

- Vitamin D is needed so the body can properly absorb calcium. Vitamin D is manufactured within the body as a result of exposure to sunlight. It can be obtained by eating eggs, some fish and butter, or by taking cod liver oil.

- Magnesium is important so the body can use vitamin D and retain calcium. It can be obtained by eating leafy green vegetables, whole grains, nuts and seeds, beans, and eggs. High phosphorus intake causes the body to become magnesium deficient. Soft drinks are very high in phosphorus.

- Boron helps the body retain calcium and magnesium. It can be obtained by eating leafy green vegetables, especially alfalfa, kelp, spinach, lettuce, and cabbage, and from apples and beans.

- Silicon is important for formation of the soft tissue in bone that keeps bones flexible instead of becoming brittle. Silicon can be obtained by eating grains with fiber, especially brown rice, oats, and barley, as well as many fruits and vegetables. The herbs horsetail and hemp nettle are also good sources of silicon.

- Vitamin C contributes to collagen formation in bones. Vitamin C can be obtained by eating leafy green vegetables, cauliflower, tomatoes, fruits, and berries. Smoking depletes the body of vitamin C.

- Hydrochloric acid (HCl) is important for the body to absorb calcium. HCl is naturally produced by the stomach, but production appears to diminish as we get older. Taking antacids, stress, and anxiety all reduce HCl production within the stomach.

IS IT POSSIBLE TO GET ENOUGH OF THESE VITAMINS AND MINERALS FROM FOOD INTAKE OR ARE SUPPLEMENTS NECESSARY?

Unfortunately, even under ideal circumstances, most women in the U.S. have difficulty consuming and assimilating enough nutrients from food alone. Therefore, preventing and treating osteoporosis usually requires more than a good diet, although adequate nutrition is very important because it provides balanced nutrients to the body.

A good multiple vitamin/mineral supplement is recommended for most menopausal and postmenopausal women for maintaining optimal overall health, especially the health of their bones.

HOW DOES A WOMAN KNOW WHICH SUPPLEMENTS TO TAKE FOR GOOD BONE HEALTH?

Selecting a nutritional supplement can be confusing because there are so many available, with varying combinations and quantities of nutrients. Since every person's genetic makeup, diet, and lifestyle differs, each individual must assess her own supplemental needs. There are numerous books that address diet and nutrition that may be helpful.

The following basic guidelines for daily supplemental intake have been shown to contribute to good bone health and fall within the safe ranges for most women. Do not exceed safe levels without the advice of a healthcare professional you trust. It may be beneficial for you discuss this list with your physician or to seek

133

the assistance of a healthcare professional with nutritional training.

Minerals: calcium, 500 to 1200 mg; magnesium, 250 to 600 mg; zinc, 10 to 30 mg; manganese, 5 to 20 mg; boron, 1 to 3 mg; silicon, 1 to 2 mg; copper, 1 to 2 mg; strontium, 0.5 to 3 mg.

Vitamins: vitamin C, 100 to 1000 mg; vitamin D, 100 to 400 IU; vitamin B-6, 5 to 50 mg; folic acid, 0.5 to 5 mg; vitamin K, 100 to 500 mcg.

WHEN IS THE BEST TIME OF DAY TO TAKE SUPPLEMENTS?

Supplements are best utilized by the body when they are ingested as food would be, in small amounts a few times a day, rather than all at one time. It is better to take most supplements with food, but others are best taken between meals. There are usually instructions on the containers if this is important.

Often mineral supplements are best taken at night or between meals because it may be difficult for the body to absorb calcium in particular when it is ingested with any of the following: excessive dietary fiber or cooked cereals and grains, spinach, squash, rhubarb, parsley, beets, and beans; caffeine in coffee, tea, sodas, or chocolate; and especially with antacids.

IS IT SAFE TO TAKE SUPPLEMENTS WHILE TAKING PRESCRIPTION MEDICATIONS?

Some nutritional supplements can alter the effects of prescription medications within the body. You need to ask your physician if the quantities of nutritional supplements you plan to take are safe with your prescription medications.

ARE THERE HERBS THAT CAN BE TAKEN FOR GOOD BONE HEALTH?

Because herbs are derived from plants, they do have nutritional value. As with all nutritional supplements, caution is needed when taking herbs. Many herbs are potent and can have a strong affect on your body. It is best to take herbs in small quantities and with the advice of a healthcare professional with a knowledge of herbs.

Some mineral/vitamin formulations also contain herbs, and health food stores carry herbal combinations specifically formulated for good bone health. The following herbs may be included:

- Black walnut contains silica.
- Comfrey contains calcium and phosphorus.
- Horsetail and rue strengthen bones.
- Oat straw is high in silica and calcium.
- Queen of the meadow contains vitamin D.
- Skullcap contains calcium and magnesium.
- White oak bark and marshmallow contain calcium.

ARE TUMS® A GOOD SOURCE OF CALCIUM?

Taking Tums has been suggested as a good source of calcium, however there is some controversy about this. While a Tums tablet does contain 200 mg of calcium carbonate, their purpose is to reduce stomach acids (HCl), which slows down digestion, and is said to reduce calcium absorption by the body.

Supplemental calcium alone is not a good preventive measure for osteoporosis. A well-rounded supplemental program is most effective.

Avoid antacids that contain aluminum, which is detrimental to a woman's bone health. Tums do not contain aluminum.

WHY IS ALUMINUM BAD FOR THE BONES?

Aluminum leaches calcium from the body, disturbing your calcium balance. Besides avoiding antacids containing aluminum, avoid cooking in aluminum containers, especially highly acidic foods such as tomatoes and tomato sauces.

It is recommended that you eliminate antiperspirants containing aluminum.

IS ALCOHOL CONSUMPTION BAD FOR THE BONES?

It is well documented that there is a high incidence of osteoporosis in male alcoholics because alcohol affects the liver's metabolism of calcium and vitamin D. Although similar studies have not been conducted with groups of women, it is assumed that the conclusions would be the same.

Moderate consumption of alcohol is a subject of some debate. Some studies suggest that moderate daily alcohol intake is beneficial to otherwise healthy individuals. Other studies conclude that any alcohol consumption is not good for the body. Everyone agrees that excessive consumption of alcohol is toxic to the body.

WHY IS WEIGHT-BEARING EXERCISE IMPORTANT FOR GOOD BONE HEALTH?

Weight-bearing exercise benefits your bones and muscles as well as providing the overall health benefits derived from regular moderate exercise. Strong muscles provide better support for your bones. Although they're not sure why, studies have shown that moderate weight-bearing exercise causes bones to become stronger.

People who are right-handed and use that hand more often usually have slightly larger bones in their right hand and arm. Astronauts who have lived in a weightless environment for extended periods of time have been shown to experience bone loss.

DOES WORKING OUT AT THE GYM, RIDING A BICYCLE, OR SWIMMING EVERY DAY KEEP BONES STRONG?

Bicycling and swimming are not weight-bearing exercises that build and strengthen bones, although they may be beneficial for the body in other ways. It is best to avoid excessive aerobic exercise that may lead to low body fat, which has an effect on hormonal balances in the body and is not beneficial for your bones. Many women athletes, such as marathon runners, ballerinas, and gymnasts, stop menstruating altogether even before they reach menopausal age due to low body fat.

WHAT'S THE BEST EXERCISE FOR KEEPING BONES HEALTHY?

Any routine, moderate weight-bearing exercise is beneficial. Although there's no best way, walking may be the easiest form of exercise for most people. Walking outdoors for one hour, two to three times a week is beneficial not only for your bones, it is good for your heart and your emotional well-being as well. Outdoor exercise during the day is an added benefit because the body manufactures vitamin D in response to sunlight exposure.

DOES STRESS NEGATIVELY AFFECT A WOMAN'S BONES?

Just as too much stress negatively affects the entire body, it is bad for the bones. The glands secrete hormones that regenerate and renew the body when it is in balance. When the mind tells the body it can't handle stress, the glands are stimulated to release extra hormones in an attempt to regain balance within the body. Stress that is not managed and controlled can further disturb the hormonal balance in a woman during menopause.

In turn, the body needs more nutritional support and quickly utilizes the nutrients available to it. If adequate nutrients are not made available to the body through food intake and supplements, the body will draw nutrients from its warehouses, often from the bones. As a result, stress can cause your body to be depleted of its nutrient supply and add to bone deterioration.

All of this can lead to enhanced hormonal imbalances, as well as vitamin, mineral, and nutritional deficiencies in the body that can lead to osteoporosis.

Chapter 6 offers suggestions for stress reduction and management.

WHY IS CIGARETTE SMOKING BAD FOR THE BONES?

Smokers generally enter menopause at a younger age than non-smokers. Early menopause is a high risk factor for developing osteoporosis. Thin women smokers are at greater risk.

There is substantial evidence linking cadmium exposure to bone disease. Cadmium is a toxic metallic element found in high concentrations in tobacco smoke. When breathed into the lungs, it easily enters the bloodstream of your body.

The effect of second-hand smoke on the bones of nonsmokers is a matter of heated debate.

Studies have shown that nutrient-deficient animals are more susceptible to the damaging effects of cadmium and that nutritional supplements buffered the toxic effects to some degree. Thin, nutrient-deficient women smokers are at triple risk for developing osteoporosis.

WHAT OTHER ENVIRONMENTAL-TOXIN OR HEAVY-METAL EXPOSURE INCREASES A WOMAN'S RISK OF OSTEOPOROSIS?

Exposure to heavy metals and environmental toxins may increase your risk of osteoporosis by leaching calcium and vitamin D from your body. Avoid:

- Exposure to aluminum in antiperspirants, antacids, cookware, some baking powder, food and beverage containers, children's aspirin, air conditioning.
- Exposure to tin in cans used for food packaging.
- Cadmium in cigarette smoke.
- Fluoride, chlorine, and other toxins in drinking water.
- Electric blankets, nonfiltered computer screens, and fluorescent lights.

DOES TAKING PRESCRIPTION MEDICATIONS INCREASE A WOMAN'S RISK OF OSTEOPOROSIS?

There is evidence that your risk of developing osteoporosis may increase if you take prescription medications, especially the following:

- Glucocorticosteroids such as cortisone and prednisone over an extended period of time interferes with bone remodeling, absorption of calcium, and retention of potassium.

- Thyroid medication over extended periods of time may increase your risk for developing osteoporosis. Although there is contradictory information coming from studies of women taking thyroid medication, it is a fact that interaction of the thyroid with the other glands of the body is important for bone remodeling. Medications that affect the thyroid functions within the body will also affect the bones.

- Antibiotics on a regular basis destroy beneficial bacteria in the intestines that is needed for adequate absorption of nutrients. When taking antibiotics, you can reestablish beneficial bacteria in the body by eating yogurt with active cultures or by taking acidophilus supplements available at health food stores.

- Laxatives and diuretics on a regular basis interfere with calcium absorption and may deplete the body of other essential minerals such as magnesium and potassium.

Estrogen replacement is also prescription medication and deserves the same attention to side effects and precautions as any other medical treatment program. Some studies have shown that taking estrogen without added progesterone does reduce bone loss, but your bones may become more brittle.

Any medication could put you at higher risk for developing osteoporosis. Discuss with your physician the side effects of over-the-counter medications as well as necessary prescription medications, and the medications' interaction with your diet and nutritional supplements, as well as a regular exercise program.

WHY ARE WOMEN WITH EATING DISORDERS,
SUCH AS BULIMIA, ANOREXIA NERVOSA,
OR SERIOUS LOSS OF APPETITE AT HIGH RISK
FOR DEVELOPING OSTEOPOROSIS?

Any eating disorder or severe loss of appetite can lead to extreme nutritional deficiencies within the body that may lead to osteoporosis. Eating disorders can also result in permanent damage to the body in other ways, with the consequences in extreme cases being disability or death.

DOES FLUORIDE IN THE DRINKING WATER MAKE BONES STRONGER?

At one time fluoride was thought to be an effective treatment for osteoporosis, and indeed fluoride does seem to encourage bone building. However later studies indicate that fluoride therapy for osteoporosis was not as effective as first believed for preventing fractures, because although bone mass increased, the bones were dry and brittle, not strong and flexible.

Although studies indicate that fluoride may be beneficial for the dental health of children, there is no proof that fluoride has the same benefits for the teeth of older people.

DOES CALCITONIN PREVENT BONE LOSS?

Calcitonin, a hormone produced by the thyroid gland, seems important to bone and calcium metabolism by slowing down the activity of osteoclasts, the cells that break down old bone, therefore preventing osteoporosis. There is a theory that exercise causes the thyroid gland to release calcitonin.

It is also believed that hormonal changes in a woman's body during pregnancy increases her calcitonin. Studies show that women who have had children appear to enter menopause with greater bone mass than women who have never given birth to a child. In addition, during pregnancy a woman's progesterone levels increase dramatically. Progesterone stimulates osteoblasts, the cells that build new bone.

IS CALCITONIN THERAPY USED TO TREAT OSTEOPOROSIS?

Calcitonin therapy has been used to inhibit bone loss in women with breast cancer, who have completed menopause naturally or through ovarian failure or removal and who cannot take estrogen because it appears to stimulate breast tumor growth.

How Does HRT
Affect Your Breasts?

The effects of *HRT* on a woman's breasts are a controversial subject with varying opinions and results from numerous studies. The decision to take *HRT* is especially serious for a woman with a high risk of breast cancer. A woman's risk factors for developing breast problems may be genetic and have been shown to be influenced by her dietary habits and whether or not she is taking *HRT.* Monitoring the conditions of your breasts is very important while taking *HRT*

DOES TAKING ESTROGEN CAUSE BREAST CANCER?

Estrogen is known to stimulate all the cells in the body, especially the breasts. Although it does not cause cancer, it may promote the growth of cancer cells that already exist within a woman's body, or of cancer cells that may develop while a woman is taking *HRT.*

A link has been made between *HRT* and an increased risk of breast cancer, with long-term use of estrogen doubling a woman's chances of developing the disease. A woman with a personal history of breast problems is usually advised not to take *HRT.* And a woman with an intense fear of breast cancer may elect not to take *HRT* unless the benefits strongly outweigh her anxiety created by the fear.

ARE A WOMAN'S CHANCES OF GETTING BREAST CANCER INCREASED BY TAKING HRT?

Whether taking *HRT* increases a woman's chances of developing breast cancer is controversial. During the 1980s several studies showed a slight increase in breast cancer risk for women taking *HRT*, but those findings were attributed to the higher doses of estrogen prescribed at that time.

Still, a recent six-year study of 23,244 Swedish women over 35 who were taking various types of estrogen found that the women had a 10 percent increase in breast cancer. The study also concluded that the longer a woman takes estrogen, the higher her risk, with women taking estrogen for nine years or longer being 70 percent more likely to develop breast cancer.

Other studies say women taking natural progesterone or progestins along with estrogen have no increased risk of breast cancer.

DOES TAKING PROGESTINS OR NATURAL PROGESTERONE WITH ESTROGEN PROTECT A WOMAN AGAINST BREAST CANCER?

Often progestins or natural progesterone are not considered a necessary ingredient of *HRT* if a woman does not have her uterus, because they are predominantly protective to the uterine lining and adding them can reduce the benefits of estrogen to the cardiovascular system. But preliminary studies indicate taking progestins or natural progesterone along with estrogen can be protective against breast cancer.

WHY DO SOME STUDIES CONCLUDE ONE THING AND OTHERS SAY SOMETHING ELSE?

The types and dosages of hormones taken, as well as the length of time they are taken seem to be the varying factors in the studies.

142

HOW DO THE TYPES, DOSAGES, AND LENGTH OF TIME A WOMAN TAKES HRT AFFECT HER RISKS OF BREAST CANCER?

Depending on a woman's personal risk factors, the best data available at present appears to indicate that long-term use of *HRT* in moderately high doses contributes somewhat to a woman's increase in breast cancer risk. Lower doses for a short period of time seem to carry no measurable risk. Lower doses of *HRT* for long periods of time have not been studied adequately enough to draw specific conclusions.

Some types of estrogen appear to be potentially more harmful than others. The potent dosages of estradiol are confirmed by most studies to significantly increase a woman's breast cancer risk. This may be why estradiol is not widely used in the U.S. The other stronger synthetic estrogens appear to be the most harmful as well. Generally, they are no longer prescribed for *HRT*, but are taken in birth control pills.

WHAT TYPES OF ESTROGEN ARE LESS HARMFUL TO A WOMAN'S BREAST HEALTH?

Most naturally-derived estrogens are considered to have a lower breast cancer risk. Phytoestrogen (plant-derived estrogen), called estriol, is said to actually protect a woman against breast cancer.

WHY IS ESTRIOL NOT PRESCRIBED MORE OFTEN TO PROTECT A WOMAN'S BREASTS?

Although estriol is widely used in Europe without problems, it has not undergone the scientific blind studies considered proof of its effectiveness and safety in the U.S. Estriol is the weakest form of natural estrogen prescribed for *HRT*. Often it does not have the same immediate results for the discomforts of menopause when given in the same dosages as other types of estrogen. *Premarin*, the conjugated estrogen often prescribed for *HRT*, will usually

143

alleviate hot flashes when taken in dosages of 0.6 to 1.25 mg, however estriol usually needs to be taken in dosages of 2 to 4 mg to have the same effect.

The higher dosage requirements of estriol are a cause of concern for many physicians. Also, it is not known if estriol has the same beneficial effects as other types of estrogen on a woman's bone health and cardiovascular system.

WHY DOES ESTRIOL HAVE A DIFFERENT EFFECT IN A WOMAN'S BREASTS THAN OTHER ESTROGENS?

The three forms of estrogen active in a woman's body are estradiol, estrone, and estriol. Estradiol is the primary estrogen the ovaries produce, estradiol is converted into estrone by the intestines, and estriol is produced in large amounts by a woman's body during pregnancy. This leads researchers to believe that there is a connection between progesterone production by the body (which is known to dramatically increase during pregnancy) and the production of estriol. Progesterone production by the ovaries usually stops before estrogen during perimenopause, resulting in irregular menstrual cycles. This leaves the body out of balance, with more estrogen. Breast problems generally are believed to be related to excessive estrogen's effect on the breasts. The anticancer effects of estriol are thought to be due to the fact that it seems to block the stimulating effect that estrone has on breast tissue. Conjugated estrogens (*Premarin*) are converted mostly to estrone in the intestinal tract.

HAVE SCIENTIFIC STUDIES BEEN CONDUCTED USING ESTRIOL?

Studies conducted twenty-five years ago using estriol showed that it inhibited breast cancer in mice. It was also discovered in a 1966 study that women with breast cancer had high levels of estrone and estradiol in their urine, but low levels of estriol, while women without breast cancer had higher estriol levels.

In a later study, published in the *Journal of the American Medical Association* in 1978, estriol was given to postmenopausal women with breast cancer and 37 percent experienced an improvement in their cancer.

DO OTHER MEDICATIONS BLOCK THE ESTROGEN EFFECT IN A WOMAN'S BODY?

Tamoxifen is a prescription drug that entirely blocks the effects of all estrogens in the body. It is being used to prevent cancer of the breasts, but it has been shown to increase a woman's risk of developing uterine cancer, so its use may not be advised for a woman with an intact uterus. The long-term effects of *Tamoxifen* on a woman's body are not known.

CAN A WOMAN WHO WANTS TO TAKE HRT FOR THE BENEFITS TO HER CARDIOVASCULAR SYSTEM AND HER BONES TAKE ESTRIOL ALONG WITH AN ESTROGEN THAT IS KNOWN TO OFFER THOSE BENEFITS?

There is a combination estrogen, called tri-estrogen, that contains 80 percent estriol with 10 percent estrone and 10 percent estradiol. When taken in a dosage of 2.5 mg for 25 day cycles with natural progesterone added at 25 to 50 mg during the last two weeks of the cycle, it is said to relieve effectively the discomforts of menopause and protect against bone deterioration, without having a negative effect on breast tissue.

It must be stressed that the use of estriol and natural progesterone have not undergone the scientific blind studies commonly recognized as proof of effectiveness by the American medical community.

WHY IS MAKING A DECISION TO TAKE HRT SO SERIOUS FOR A WOMAN WITH A BREAST CANCER RISK?

Breast cancer can quickly spread within the breast tissue and into the rest of a woman's body. Although it is considered to be one of the most curable types of cancer in women, early detection is important. Cancerous tumors of the breast tissue are often painless and hide within breast tissue.

WHAT IS CANCER?

The cells of the body are programmed like a computer to serve specific functions within the body. When the body is functioning normally, all cells remain where they belong and do only the work they are programmed to do. Cancer occurs when cells begin to move out of their assigned positions in the body and overpower other cells. No one knows exactly what causes the migration of cells that leads to cancer, but once it occurs, stimulation of the cancer cells can cause them to increase. Estradiol and estrone are believed to stimulate the growth of cancer cells that already exist or that develop in the body.

HOW DOES CANCER DEVELOP IN A WOMAN'S BREASTS?

The abnormal growth of cells in the breast usually forms a lump or a tumor. These cells may multiply, overtaking normal cells and tissue, sometimes spreading to other parts of the body. The most common form of breast cancer involves the cells of the glands and ducts. Less common forms of breast cancer start in the skin around the nipples, oil glands around hair follicles, the sweat glands, or other cells within the breast.

DO ALL WOMEN HAVE AN EQUAL CHANCE OF GETTING BREAST CANCER?

Only about 10 percent of all women get breast cancer, with women living in Canada, Denmark, England, Israel, the Netherlands, and Scotland having a slightly higher risk than women in the U.S. Women living in Asia, especially in Japan, have a lower rate of breast cancer. However, when women migrate to Hawaii or the continental U.S. from Asia, their risk of

146

breast cancer increases, which indicates an environmental or dietary link associated with breast cancer.

DOES A WOMAN WITH BREAST CANCER HAVE HIGHER LEVELS OF ESTROGEN IN HER BLOOD?

Results of several studies show higher levels of estrogen in the blood of women who have breast cancer. Women with more body fat may have an increased risk of breast cancer because they generally have higher blood-estrogen levels.

Women past menopause with apple-shaped bodies resulting in predominant upper body fat (in the waist, arms, shoulders, and nape of the neck) appear to be more likely to develop breast cancer. While women with pear-shaped bodies with fat distribution centering in the hips and thighs have a lower risk of breast cancer.

WHAT ARE THE BREAST CANCER RISK FACTORS A WOMAN NEEDS TO CONSIDER BEFORE DECIDING ON HRT?

There appears to be a genetic predisposition to breast cancer, so a woman whose female blood relatives have had breast cancer needs to be more cautious about taking *HRT,* especially a woman whose mother or sister experienced breast cancer in both breasts before menopause. This is considered hereditary breast cancer.

Hormonal factors are also said to influence a woman's risk of developing breast cancer. They include:

- Menstruation onset at an early age. Studies have shown that women who had their first menstrual period before the age of 12 have twice the risk of breast cancer than women who started menstruating at 13 or later.

- Menopause at a later age. Women who have their last menstrual period at age 45 have half the risk of developing breast cancer as women who enter menopause after 55.

- Number of years of active menstrual cycles. Women with 30

years of regular active menstruation have half the risk for developing breast cancer compared to women who have regular active menstruation for 40 years or longer.

A woman's age and the conditions of her breasts and body fat may also be factors:

- Breast cancer usually occurs in women over 40. Possibly, because after that age hormone levels change in the body, often resulting in excessive estrogen effect on the breasts.
- Being overweight after menopause. Although excess body fat in women younger than 50 does not appear to affect their risk of breast cancer, women over 60 with excess body fat have as much as an 80 percent greater chance for developing breast cancer. Although the reasons are unclear, this may be related to the fact that the body converts androgens (male hormones) in body fat to estrogen after menopause.
- Women with dense breast tissue are likelier to develop breast cancer. A mammogram is necessary to determine whether your breast tissue is dense.
- A personal history of fibrocysts in the breasts may increase a woman's chances for developing breast cancer, because fibrocysts are believed to result from excessive estrogen effect on breast tissue.

Childbearing also appears to be a factor in a woman's breast cancer risk:

- Women who have never had children have a higher risk of developing breast cancer.
- A woman giving birth to her first child later in life, after the age of 30, is at higher risk for developing breast cancer than one whose first child was born when she was 20 or younger.
- Women who breastfeed their first child for at least six months appear to have a lower risk of breast cancer.

Women who smoke cigarettes and drink alcoholic beverages are at higher risk of developing breast cancer. This may be related to the effects of these substances on the liver, which is responsible for metabolizing estrogen so that excess hormones can be excreted from the body instead of being stored in the tissues.

Studies have shown that exposure to environmental toxins such as pesticides, especially DDT, increases a woman's risk of breast cancer. Although the use of DDT was banned in 1972, it can be stored in the fatty tissues of the body for decades. Chemicals similar to DDT that are chlorine-based are still used as pesticides and in various other ways, such as in disinfectants for swimming pools and in spot removers.

Artificial menopause due to surgical removal of the ovaries reduces a woman's risk of breast cancer.

DOES HEREDITARY BREAST CANCER HAVE SPECIAL CHARACTERISTICS?

Recent studies are believed to prove that certain types of breast cancer are genetically transmitted and can come from either your mother's or your father's side of the family. That is why it is so important to give a complete medical history of both sides of your family to your doctor when deciding whether to take *HRT.*

Hereditary breast cancer occurs earlier in life, with the average age being 44, as compared to 60 or over for other women.

Hereditary breast cancer involves both breasts in about 46 percent of cases. Women having hereditary breast cancer are at higher risk for developing other cancers such as ovarian, brain, lung, colon, adrenal gland, thyroid, and leukemia.

A woman with a parent or sibling with breast cancer falls into the highest risk category. A woman with maternal or paternal grandparents, aunts, or uncles with cancer are also considered at risk, although the risk is not as high.

HOW CAN A WOMAN DETECT CHANGES IN HER BREAST AS EARLY AS POSSIBLE?

It is important for all woman to be concerned about detecting breast changes, especially while taking *HRT* and in the years just before menopause when breast cancer is more likely to occur.

Committing to three routine breast examinations gives you the best chance of detecting breast problems as early as possible:

- A monthly self-examination of your breasts.
- A breast physical examination by a healthcare professional at least once a year or more often for women who fall into a high-risk category or those with a personal history of breast problems.
- A mammogram on a regular basis.

WHAT IS A MAMMOGRAM?

A mammogram is an x ray of the breast tissue that is able to detect tumors too small to be felt in either a self-breast exam or a physical exam by your physician. The American Cancer Society encourages all women to have regular mammograms because by the time a cancerous growth in the breast is large enough to be felt in a physical exam, it may have been present for three to seven years. When detected early, breast cancer is said to have at least a 90 percent chance of being cured.

HOW OFTEN DOES A WOMAN NEED A MAMMOGRAM?

The American Cancer Society suggests a woman have mammograms as follows:

- A woman with a high incidence of breast cancer in direct female blood relatives may choose to have her first mammogram as early as age 25. At the very least, she needs to discuss this with her physician.
- A woman between 35 and 40 who has not already done so needs a mammogram as a baseline for comparison of all future mammograms, as well as for detection of early breast cancer.
- A woman between 40 and 49 is advised to have a

mammogram every one or two years, depending on her personal medical history and risk factors.

- A woman is advised to have a mammogram once a year when she is over 50 or if she is over 40 and falls into a high-risk category for breast cancer.

WHEN DOES A WOMAN NEED TO HAVE HER PHYSICIAN EXAMINE HER BREASTS?

A woman taking *HRT* needs to have her breasts routinely examined by her physician during her annual physical checkup. Because small lumps within the breasts can easily be missed during this exam if it is rushed, make sure your physician takes the time to be thorough.

Whenever a woman detects breast changes of any kind during a self-breast exam, an additional physician breast exam is absolutely necessary and needs to be performed as soon as possible.

HOW OFTEN DOES A WOMAN NEED TO DO A BREAST SELF-EXAM

Every woman needs to perform a breast self-examination at least once a month. Often a breast lump is found by a woman herself, not by her physician. Although early cancer is usually painless, while other types of breast problems, such as fibrocysts, are painful to the touch, any lump a woman discovers in her breasts or in her armpit needs to be reported to her physician immediately.

It is best to schedule routine breast self-exams with yourself on a date that is easily remembered, such as the first or last day of the month. If you are on cyclic *HRT* and have found a routine change in your breasts during the month, you may want to examine yourself two times a month, at a time when your breasts feel unaffected by the hormones, as well as during the time when the breasts are routinely reacting to the hormones.

DO A WOMAN'S BREASTS RESPOND TO HRT THE SAME WAY THEY RESPOND TO THE NATURAL MENSTRUAL CYCLE?

Women taking cyclic *HRT*, as described in chapter 2, may see or feel slight changes in their breasts during the month similar to the natural cyclic release of hormones by the ovaries. These effects vary depending on the type and dosages of hormones taken.

Breast reactions while taking *HRT* may be considered routine when they occur at the same time every month, with some women on *HRT* experiencing general breast tenderness and sensitivity or a slight swelling of the breasts all the time.

If you notice breast changes when you first start taking *HRT* it is always best to discuss these changes with your physician. An adjustment in your type of *HRT* or your dosage may be needed.

WHY DO A WOMAN'S BREASTS CHANGE DURING A NATURAL MENSTRUAL CYCLE?

After ovulation, when the ovaries produce increased amounts of progesterone, a woman's body is preparing for the possibility of pregnancy. As a result, a woman often experiences premenstrual breast tenderness, some swelling of breast cells or fluid in the breasts.

WHAT DOES A WOMAN NEED TO LOOK FOR WHEN SHE DOES A BREAST SELF-EXAM?

A woman needs to look at her breasts as well as feel her breasts during her monthly self-exam.

Standing before a mirror, look to see if the size, color, or shape of your breasts has changed in any way, if either breast has taken on a shape different from the other, if there are any obvious lumps or areas of thickened breast tissue, or if there is any crustiness or scaliness on your breasts, especially around the nipples. Raise your hands over your head and look to see if your nipples are inverted or if your breasts have developed any new dimples. If any of these changes or conditions exist, it is necessary to consult your physician right away.

After examining your breasts in the mirror, lie down on a bed to feel for lumps in your breasts. Applying a little oil to your breast during this procedure can make it more comfortable.

Examine one breast at a time, folding the same arm over your head to flatten the breast as much as possible. Using the pads of the fingers on your opposite hand, slowly make small circular motions around your breast, beginning at the nipple and working outward, covering the entire breast. Feel your breasts for lumps that are harder than normal breast tissue or lumps that do not move freely when you touch them.

Then move to your armpit. You may feel lymph nodes that are normally soft, move freely, and are not painful. If your lymph nodes are firm and do not move freely, report this as well as any suspicious lumps in your breasts to your physician immediately.

Finally, gently squeeze each nipple to see if there is any blood or fluid discharge. A pink, bloody, clear yellow, or watery discharge needs to be reported to your physician as soon as possible. A slight milky discharge can be caused by medications you are taking or from childbirth, even years earlier. Still, report it to your physician.

ARE ALL THE LUMPS A WOMAN MIGHT FIND IN HER BREASTS CANCEROUS?

Very often the lumps a woman finds during a breast self exam are fibrocysts not cancer. Usually, lumps that are harder than normal breast tissue and do not move freely are more suspicious. However, it is always best to report any breast changes or lumps to your doctor. While approximately 10 percent of women develop breast cancer, as many as 40-to-60 percent experience fibrocystic breasts.

WHAT ARE FIBROCYSTS OF THE BREAST?

Fibrocysts of the breast is a broad term that refers to approximately 50 different benign breast conditions. When a woman's breast feels lumpy and it is referred to as cystic, she may also be told she has fibrocystic breast disease, although it isn't really a disease. Some fibrocysts are simply variations of normal breast tissue, but others are more suspicious and deserve closer attention. In true cystic breast disease, a cyst in a woman's breast becomes prominent and fills with fluid. They are often accompanied by breast tenderness and some women experience intense pain from fibrocysts of the breasts.

Fibrocystic breast disease is common in perimenopausal and postmenopausal women.

DO FIBROCYSTS TURN INTO BREAST CANCER?

Some studies say fibrocysts do not turn into breast cancer, while others say women with fibrocysts have a two-to-five-times greater risk of developing breast cancer.

DOES TAKING HRT HAVE AN EFFECT ON FIBROCYSTS OF THE BREAST?

It is believed that fibrocysts of the breasts are related to low progesterone levels and excessive estrogen effect on the breasts. Therefore, the conclusion would be that taking a combination estrogen/progestin *HRT* would be more beneficial for a woman who has experienced fibrocysts of the breasts.

Studies using natural progesterone have shown that it is very effective in relieving the pain of fibrocysts and may decrease their development.

WHAT DO DOCTORS RECOMMEND FOR THE TREATMENT OF FIBROCYSTIC BREASTS?

Usually, a physician will suggest that a lump of any kind be biopsied to determine that is not cancer. Once it is determined that a lump is a fibrocyst, the treatment can include several things. Hormones may be suggested to balance the estrogen and progesterone effects on the breast.

Diuretics may be advised because fibrocysts often are filled with fluid. Pain medication can offer relief when the fibrocysts are extremely painful, and dietary changes are usually suggested.

HOW DOES A WOMAN'S DIET AFFECT FIBROCYSTS OF THE BREASTS?

Caffeine and chocolate intake has been linked to fibrocysts of the breast. Coffee, some tea, cola drinks with caffeine, and chocolate contain substances belonging to a family of chemicals called methylxanthines. Studies have shown that totally eliminating products containing these chemicals will usually eliminate fibrocysts of the breasts. Cutting down on foods and beverages containing these chemicals is not good enough, they need to be completely eliminated from the diet. Once the fibrocysts clear up, if a woman starts to eat and drink these foods and beverages again, the condition usually returns. However, there can be side effects when suddenly stopping caffeine intake altogether. Chapter 6 contains more information about caffeine intake and stopping.

A high-fat diet has been associated with fibrocysts of the breast by increasing body fat. Androgens in body fat are converted to estrogen by the body, contributing to an estrogen-progesterone imbalance and increasing the estrogen effect on the breasts.

Studies also show that intake of 600 IU of vitamin E daily, along with B complex and the trace mineral selenium results in an improvement in fibrocystic breast problems in 75 percent of women.

DOES A WOMAN'S DIETARY FAT INTAKE AFFECT HER RISK OF BREAST CANCER?

Breast cancer appears to develop in stages over a number of years and may be influenced by diet, especially saturated fats. Studies of the correlation between dietary fat intake and breast cancer have led to the conclusion that a high saturated fat diet increases a woman's risk of developing breast cancer and causes existing breast cancer to be more difficult to control.

It has been reported that a diet high in saturated fat seems to contribute to benign (noncancerous) breast tumors changing to cancer. Active breast cancer has been shown to grow faster and spread farther in women with a high-fat diet, especially older women.

WHAT FOODS ARE HIGH IN SATURATED FATS THAT A WOMAN MIGHT WANT TO AVOID?

The foods highest in saturated fat include animal fats contained in meat, high-fat cheeses, whole milk, butter, coconut oil, and any oil that is solid at room temperature.

DO OTHER DIETARY FACTORS AFFECT A WOMAN'S RISK OF DEVELOPING BREAST CANCER?

Numerous studies have shown various dietary factors that affect a woman's chances of developing breast cancer, including:

- In 1991, the *International Journal of Cancer* advised that a high intake of dietary fiber, vitamin C, and beta carotene decreases a woman's risk of postmenopausal breast cancer.

- Other studies have concluded that low thyroid activity due to inadequate dietary intake of iodine can increase a woman's risk of developing breast cancer. Women who live in Japan and Iceland, where iodine is adequately consumed in seafood and seaweed, have a lower incidence of breast cancer.

- Women with cancer had lower-than-normal blood levels of the trace mineral selenium. Soil with low levels of selenium correlate to areas of the world where women have the highest cancer incidence. However, selenium can be toxic when taken in excess, with no more than 200 mcg daily being the upper limit of intake.

- Because a woman's liver function affects metabolism of estrogen in the body, a healthy liver activity is said to reduce a woman's risk of breast cancer. Liver activity may be enhanced with adequate intake of B-complex vitamins, vitamin C, and the trace minerals zinc, copper, manganese, and selenium.

• Specific foods can reduce the body's sensitivity to carcinogens, including cruciferous vegetables such as broccoli, cabbage, and cauliflower. They are believed to have anti-breast cancer elements, called phytochemical indole-3-carbinol (I3C), which deactivate estrogens that stimulate the growth of breast cancer.

CHAPTER 11

How Does HRT Affect Your Cardiovascular System?

Estrogen can be beneficial to the cardiovascular health of a woman after menopause by lowering her blood cholesterol. However, taking a progestin along with estrogen may diminish these benefits somewhat. Your chances of developing cardiovascular disease after menopause can be significantly affected by heredity, diet, and lifestyle.

WHY IS A WOMAN'S CARDIOVASCULAR HEALTH AN IMPORTANT CONSIDERATION WHEN DECIDING WHETHER TO TAKE HRT?

The incidence of cardiovascular disease increases significantly in women after menopause. Before age 50, men are six to seven times likelier than women to have heart attacks. After 60, a woman's likelihood of heart attack seems to become about equal with a man's.

WHY DOES HRT HAVE DIFFERENT EFFECTS ON A WOMAN'S CARDIOVASCULAR SYSTEM THAN BIRTH CONTROL PILLS?

Although both *HRT* and birth control pills contain estrogen and progestins, the types and dosages of these hormones are different. The estrogens in birth control pills are usually stronger synthetic estrogens that stop ovulation. The estrogens in *HRT* are usually naturally derived estrogens and their dosages are much smaller.

Further, birth control pills often contain stronger progestins derived from testosterone, while the progestins in *HRT* are usually naturally derived.

Consequently, the hormones in birth control pills and those in *HRT* seem to have different effects on a woman's cardiovascular system.

WHAT ARE THE DIFFERENCES IN THE EFFECTS OF HRT AND BIRTH CONTROL PILLS ON A WOMAN'S CARDIOVASCULAR SYSTEM?

Taking the birth control pill is known to increase a woman's risk of developing dangerous blood clots (thrombophlebitis), but the estrogens in *HRT* increase a woman's blood clotting abilities only slightly. That increase is considered beneficial because when a woman goes through menopause her blood does not clot as easily as it once did.

Taking the birth control pill has been shown to potentially increase a woman's risk of high blood pressure (hypertension), while the estrogen in *HRT* appears to lower a woman's blood pressure. Even so, a woman who is likely to experience hypertension needs to have her blood pressure monitored more closely when she takes *HRT*.

Women with diabetes are sometimes advised not to take the birth control pill because it has an adverse effect on the body's sugar metabolism. However, the estrogen in *HRT* does not have that same effect in a woman's body.

WHAT ARE THE LONG-TERM EFFECTS OF ESTROGEN ON A WOMAN'S CARDIOVASCULAR SYSTEM?

Studies have shown that the longer a woman takes estrogen, the more it reduces her risk of cardiovascular disease by positively affecting her blood cholesterol levels. Estrogen is also believed to relax the blood vessels, easing heart function.

HOW DOES ESTROGEN BENEFIT A WOMAN'S BLOOD CHOLESTEROL LEVELS?

Estrogen has been shown to protect a woman against heart attack by raising the levels of HDL (high density lipoprotein), good cholesterol, in the blood while lowering LDL (low density lipoprotein), bad cholesterol. HDL collects fat and cholesterol in the blood within envelopes, which allows them to be carried out of the bloodstream, instead of breaking down and being deposited on the artery walls. LDL breaks down more easily and deposits fat on artery walls.

ARE THE PROGESTINS TAKEN ALONG WITH ESTROGEN BENEFICIAL FOR A WOMAN'S CARDIOVASCULAR SYSTEM?

Although medical opinions differ, progestins are generally believed to diminish the positive effects of estrogen on the cardiovascular system. Thus, a women without an intact uterus who takes *HRT* is prescribed unopposed estrogen (estrogen without progestins), as the progestins are needed primarily to protect the uterus.

Progestins may contribute to sodium retention in some women, possibly leading to hypertension.

ARE THE EFFECTS OF NATURAL PROGESTERONE ON A WOMAN'S CARDIOVASCULAR SYSTEM THE SAME AS THE EFFECTS OF PROGESTINS?

Natural progesterone has been shown to be protective against high blood pressure because it has a natural diuretic effect on the body, reducing fluid retention. Natural progesterone is also said to normalize blood clotting.

IF A WOMAN STILL HAS HER UTERUS, IS IT ALWAYS NECESSARY FOR HER TO TAKE A PROGESTIN OR NATURAL PROGESTERONE ALONG WITH ESTROGEN?

Usually, a progestin or natural progesterone is prescribed along with estrogen for a woman with an intact uterus, however, this is something a woman needs to discuss with her physician. All her risk factors need to be considered to determine what type of hormones she may want and need to take, as well as what dosages may be best.

DOES EVERY WOMAN NEED ESTROGEN TO MAINTAIN GOOD CARDIOVASCULAR HEALTH?

As estrogen levels diminish in a woman's body during and after menopause, it is believed that her LDL creeps upward, her HDL declines, and her risk of developing cardiovascular disease increases. However, there are other factors besides estrogen production that either add to or reduce a woman's risk of cardiovascular disease after menopause.

DOES A WOMEN WHO HAS EARLY MENOPAUSE HAVE A HIGHER RISK OF CARDIOVASCULAR DISEASE?

Studies indicate that women who have early menopause, either naturally or because of surgical removal of their ovaries, are at higher risk of cardiovascular disease.

BESIDES MENOPAUSE, WHAT ARE THE OTHER CARDIOVASCULAR RISK FACTORS A WOMAN NEEDS TO CONSIDER WHEN DECIDING ABOUT HRT?

A woman is at higher risk of developing coronary artery disease or having a stroke when she:

- has a family history of cardiovascular disease or stroke before the age of 55
- has high blood pressure
- has elevated cholesterol levels, especially LDL (bad) cholesterol
- smokes cigarettes
- is overweight
- is diabetic.

WHAT IS CORONARY ARTERY DISEASE?

Coronary artery disease is usually caused by atherosclerosis, narrowing or blockage of arteries that supply blood to the heart or brain, decreasing the supply of oxygen and nutrients to those muscles. Lack of oxygen and nutrient-rich blood to the heart can lead to chest pains and heart attack. Lack of oxygen and nutrient-rich blood to the brain can cause stroke.

WHAT CAUSES THE ARTERIES TO BECOME NARROW OR BLOCKED?

Narrowing or blockage of the arteries, caused by atherosclerosis, is a result of plaques (cholesterol and other fatty substances) gradually collecting on the inner walls of the arteries. The slow build-up of plaque on artery walls appears to begin early in life, but women are usually protected from blockage of the arteries before menopause because of their natural estrogen production.

A partial blockage of the coronary arteries may result in angina pectoris, severe chest pains that are usually a warning sign that heart attack could result unless diet adjustments or medical treatment intervenes to relieve the blockage. A narrowing of the major arteries supplying blood to the lower body can cause pains in the legs during exercise.

WHAT DO CHEST PAINS CAUSED BY PARTIALLY BLOCKED ARTERIES FEEL LIKE?

Chest pains called angina pectoris are caused by partially blocked arteries, usually characterized by severe crushing pains in the chest below the breast bone, often with pain radiating into the left arm. Sometimes it feels like heartburn that cannot be relieved by antacids. However, chest pains of any kind are not to be dismissed simply as heartburn or hot flashes. They need to be reported to your physician at once.

WHAT'S THE DIFFERENCE BETWEEN ANGINA AND A HEART ATTACK?

A heart attack occurs when a coronary artery or one of its branches becomes blocked to the point that its supply of blood to the heart stops. That causes the area of the heart not getting blood to die and become scarred.

If a major heart attack occurs, death can result.

WHAT HAPPENS WHEN A STROKE OCCURS?

A stroke is a rupture in a blocked artery supplying blood to the brain. It can result in the loss of various bodily functions, depending on the part of the brain deprived of blood. A woman may lose the strength of grip in her hands; she may lose her balance, becoming unsteady on her feet; or she may lose control of her speech, her words becoming slurred.

When a major stroke occurs, sudden death can result.

ARE THERE SPECIFIC RISK FACTORS ASSOCIATED WITH STROKES?

A woman with high blood pressure is more likely to have a stroke.

WHAT DETERMINES A WOMAN'S BLOOD PRESSURE?

A woman's blood pressure is measured by two factors: the amount of blood being pumped throughout the cardiovascular system and the tightness of the blood vessels through which the blood is being pumped by the heart.

WHAT CAN A WOMAN DO TO LOWER HER BLOOD PRESSURE?

Because high blood pressure (hypertension) can lead to heart attack and stroke, it is important to have your physician monitor your blood pressure, especially after menopause. There are various ways your health care professional might suggest you can reduce your blood pressure:

- HRT may decrease your blood pressure.

- Prescription medication may be needed if you have severe hypertension.

- Diet changes are extremely effective at reducing high blood pressure and eliminating excess body fat, especially:

  - Reducing fat, sugar, and sodium intake.

  - Increasing daily potassium intake by drinking orange juice, eating raw fresh vegetables, tomatoes, or apples.

  - Using a potassium-based salt substitute such as *Morton Salt Substitute, Nu-Salt,* or *No Salt.* However, a woman with kidney problems needs to check with her physician before using these products.

  - Taking a calcium, magnesium, and vitamin D supplement to restore mineral balance to the body and relax blood vessels.

  - Avoiding crash diets to lose weight as they often deplete the body of vital nutrients.

  - Avoiding soft water purified by using sodium. Drink bottled water instead.

A woman with extremely high blood pressure or severe diabetes who needs *HRT* for other reasons may be advised to use the estrogen patch.

WHY WOULD USING THE ESTROGEN PATCH BE BETTER FOR A WOMAN WITH HIGH BLOOD PRESSURE OR DIABETES?

When estrogen is taken orally it passes through the liver before entering the general blood circulation. If estrogen enters the circulation through the skin, its effect on the body appears to be the same except it passes through the liver last, causing its effect on the liver to be greatly reduced.

This would benefit a woman with severe hypertension or with a diabetic condition, because one of the liver's functions is to convert and store sugar to be used by the body. The liver produces a protein called renin substrate that affects blood pressure.

However, when the patch is used instead of oral hormones, the benefits of estrogen on blood cholesterol levels are also reduced. Estrogen stimulates production of cholesterol by the liver, usually increasing HDL cholesterol and decreasing LDL cholesterol.

HOW DOES A WOMAN KNOW WHAT HER CHOLESTEROL LEVELS ARE?

A blood test will determine your blood cholesterol levels during your extensive physical examination before you decide whether to take *HRT.* See chapter 4.

WHAT IS BLOOD CHOLESTEROL?

Cholesterol is a soft, waxy, fatty substance used by the body to manufacture hormones, bile acid, and vitamin D. It is found in every part of your body, including the nervous system, muscles, skin, liver, intestines, heart, and most other organs.

WHY ARE DIFFERENT KINDS OF CHOLESTEROL MEASURED IN THE BLOOD?

Cholesterol is transported through your body by attaching itself to lipoproteins, two types of proteins that serve different functions.

The two types of lipoproteins measured in your blood are high-density lipoprotein (HDL) and low-density lipoprotein (LDL). LDL delivers cholesterol to where it is needed in the body and deposits it there. HDL takes unneeded cholesterol from the body's cells and tissues and carries it to the liver, where it can be excreted.

The blood contains more LDL and less HDL, but these levels must fall within a normal range for you to have good cardiovascular health.

166

WHAT ARE NORMAL HDL AND LDL CHOLESTEROL RANGES?

To determine your cardiovascular health based on blood cholesterol levels, your doctor needs to have your total cholesterol level determined as well as your LDL and HDL levels. The levels of each of the three are one indication of your cardiovascular health:

- Total cholesterol count lower than 200 is considered good. A count of 200–239 borders on high risk, a count above 249 is considered high risk.

- LDL cholesterol count under 130 is considered good, 130–159 borders on high risk, and above 160 is high risk.

- HDL cholesterol count above 55 is considered good, 35–55 borders on high risk, and less than 35 is considered high.

If you divide your total cholesterol count by your HDL cholesterol count, a 4.5 or less result is good. Anything above 4.5 indicates a higher risk of cardiovascular disease.

It is better for your LDL (bad) cholesterol count to fall into a low range and your HDL (good) cholesterol count to fall into a high range, usually indicating a lower risk for cardiovascular disease.

WHAT WOULD MAKE A WOMAN'S CHOLESTEROL LEVELS EXCEED NORMAL RANGES?

The body can produce all the cholesterol it needs to function properly, so dietary cholesterol you eat may contribute to higher cholesterol levels if it cannot be carried out of the body effectively.

Even though your diet is a strong contributor to your blood cholesterol levels, it is believed there is a genetic predisposition to either healthy or unhealthy cholesterol levels, even with an ideal diet.

WHAT CAN A WOMAN DO IF HER CHOLESTEROL IS TOO HIGH?

A woman with a high total cholesterol level needs to have her HDL and LDL levels checked to see if she is high in the HDL (good) or the LDL (bad).

If your LDL cholesterol count is very high your doctor may suggest that you take medication to reduce your cholesterol, that you begin taking estrogen if you are past menopause, that you lose weight if you are overweight, or that you consume a low-cholesterol diet.

HOW MUCH DIETARY CHOLESTEROL IS IT SAFE TO EAT IN ONE DAY?

A healthy diet is one limited to no more than 300 mg of cholesterol daily, with less that 30 percent of your calories coming from fat.

The average American diet contains higher than advised levels of cholesterol, with 350–450 mg being average, and 35 to 40 percent of caloric intake coming from fat.

WHAT FOODS INCREASE A WOMAN'S CHOLESTEROL LEVELS?

A diet high in saturated fats tends to increase cholesterol levels. Saturated fats are found primarily in animal products such as meat, poultry, and whole dairy products such as cheese and butter, as well as in coconut and palm oils, and in any oils that are solid at room temperature.

WHICH FOODS BENEFIT A WOMAN'S CARDIOVASCULAR HEALTH?

Instead of saturated fatty oils use unsaturated fats, oils liquid at room temperature including olive, canola, corn, safflower, soybean, and sunflower. Increase your intake of dietary fiber, which tends to soak up cholesterol, preventing it from being absorbed into your bloodstream, and carries it out of your body.

Foods high in vitamins C, B-6, E, and magnesium are said to lower cholesterol levels, keeping the arteries clean and the blood free flowing. Foods with a natural cholesterol-lowering effect include apples, barley, beans, carrots, chili peppers, eggplant, garlic, grapefruit, lecithin from soybeans, oat bran, onions, plantains (a variety of green banana), seafood, seaweed, soybeans, spinach, yams, and yogurt.

CAN A WOMAN'S CARDIOVASCULAR HEALTH BENEFIT FROM REGULAR EXERCISE?

Routine moderate exercise benefits you in many ways, including aiding your cardiovascular health by increasing your circulation and stamina, aiding in weight loss, and reducing stress. The effects of negative stress on the body can be a significant contributor to cardiovascular problems.

ARE THERE HERBS THAT BENEFIT THE CARDIOVASCULAR SYSTEM?

The following herbs may be taken on the advice of a healthcare professional to benefit your individual cardiovascular health needs:

- Ginkgo biloba is used by millions of people in Europe and Asia because of its benefits to the cardiovascular system. It is said to improve circulation and increase the oxygen supply to the heart and other organs, to counteract the effects of angina, and to increase blood supply to the brain, thus improving memory and alertness.

- Hawthorne berries are widely used in Europe to lower cholesterol and as a heart tonic. They are said to strengthen and balance the heart, preventing or reducing irregular heart beat and protecting against oxygen deficiency.

- Ginseng is said to prevent atherosclerosis, hypertension, and to reduce cholesterol levels.

▲ ▲ ▲

How Does HRT Affect Your Pelvic Organs?

Taking estrogen after menopause can have a beneficial effect on the condition of a woman's vagina, bladder, and urinary tract, but can be detrimental to her uterine lining. Progestins or natural progesterone have a protective effect on the lining of the uterus. A woman with an intact uterus is usually advised to take a progestin or natural progesterone along with estrogen as *HRT.*

BLADDER AND URINARY TRACT

CAN TAKING HRT *STOP URINARY INCONTINENCE AND BLADDER PROBLEMS IN POSTMENOPAUSAL WOMEN?*

Taking estrogen can reduce the problem of urinary incontinence and atrophy of the bladder in postmenopausal women. Estrogen improves the capillary blood flow and nerve supply to the pelvic organs, helps tone and improve the elasticity of the tissues supporting the bladder, and thickens urethral tissue, improving a woman's ability to control the urine loss that leads to urinary incontinence.

WHY DO SOME WOMEN EXPERIENCE URINARY OR BLADDER PROBLEMS AFTER MENOPAUSE?

A woman's urinary bladder, located in the front of the pelvic cavity, sits on top of her vagina and cervix. Her urethra, the 1.5-inch tube that carries urine from the bladder out of the body, runs along the top portion of the vaginal wall, emptying just above the vaginal opening. The urethra and bladder are supported by the same estrogen-sensitive tissues as the vagina. Loss of estrogen can cause the tissues of the urinary tract and bladder to become thinner and to atrophy, making them more vulnerable to infection by organisms they were once able to resist. Recurrent bladder infections and urinary incontinence may result. In severe cases a woman's bladder and uterus may drop, causing numerous physical problems.

HOW DOES A WOMAN KNOW IF HER BLADDER AND URETHRA ARE BEGINNING TO ATROPHY?

A woman may suspect bladder or urethra atrophy if she feels a burning sensation while urinating, if she develops a need to urinate more frequently, if she feels an urgent need to urinate, if she has difficulty holding her urine, or involuntarily wets her pants. These symptoms can occur because of bladder inflammations or infections, usually accompanied by some pain, but they may also occur without infection.

DOES URINARY AND BLADDER ATROPHY FROM LOSS OF ESTROGEN AT MENOPAUSE CAUSE URINARY INCONTINENCE?

Urinary incontinence can occur before menopause as well as after. Premenopausal urinary incontinence is usually not related to lack of estrogen. Some women have an inherited tendency for weak connective tissue between the vagina and its supportive structures. More often, premenopausal urinary incontinence results from the vagina and its supportive tissues being weakened during childbirth, especially in women who have had more than one large baby or who had significant vaginal tearing.

Urinary incontinence that first occurs after menopause is usually related to loss of estrogen. Often it is a progressive condition that begins with stress incontinence.

WHAT IS STRESS INCONTINENCE?

Stress incontinence is the uncontrollable loss of urine that occurs when a woman sneezes, coughs, laughs, jumps rope, or exercises.

WHAT CAUSES A WOMAN TO HAVE STRESS INCONTINENCE AFTER MENOPAUSE?

Menopausal or postmenopausal stress incontinence is usually related to estrogen loss, when the muscle tissues surrounding the urethra become weakened and less elastic. Then, the urethral lining may be unable to control the release of urine, or the angle between the urethra and the bladder may change so urine is not prevented from dripping under sudden pressure.

Stress incontinence may also be related to emotional stress. If stress incontinence occurs suddenly after an extreme emotional upset, in time and with emotional healing, the condition may subside.

CAN TAKING ESTROGEN STOP THE LOSS OF BLADDER CONTROL FOR THE REST OF A WOMAN'S LIFE?

Taking estrogen can strongly contribute to a woman's maintaining her bladder control well into the later years. However, eventually natural aging will result in some loss of nerve supply to the bladder. A woman in her eighties may experience some loss of bladder control even if she is taking estrogen. In extreme cases of urinary incontinence or loss of bladder control, surgery may be needed.

However, if a woman regularly does the Kegel exercises, she can strengthen and tone the muscles around the bladder and rectum, improving mild stress incontinence. No one knows for sure, but starting Kegel exercises early in life and continuing them as a regular routine into later life may help you avoid developing incontinence and loss of bladder control.

HOW ARE KEGEL EXERCISES PERFORMED?

To perform the Kegel exercises, tighten the muscles around the vagina, bladder, and rectum by squeezing your vagina and but-tocks, then releasing them. Repeat this exercise 20 to 30 times several times a day. You can do them anytime and anywhere.

When you urinate, stop the flow, hold it for a few seconds, then allow it to continue.

After doing the Kegel exercises for several months, most women feel a marked improvement in the tone of their pelvic muscles. The exercises also tone the vaginal muscles and tighten the entrance to the vagina.

IS THERE ANYTHING ELSE A WOMAN CAN DO TO AVOID OR ARREST BLADDER AND URINARY TRACT INFECTION?

Bladder infections often start in the urethra, then spread to the bladder. Antibiotics taken for bladder infections can destroy the body's friendly bacteria and may lead to recurrent bladder infections, as well as to vaginal irritation and infection. Reestablishing beneficial bacteria in the body by taking acidophilus or eating yogurt with active cultures has been shown to be beneficial.

Folk remedies used for centuries to alleviate bladder infection include eating fresh cranberries or garlic and drinking cranberry juice, cherry juice, or corn silk tea.

Taking vitamin C has also been shown to be helpful in soothing and healing inflammations that cause urinary and genital ailments.

UTERUS

WHEN IS A WOMAN ADVISED NOT TO TAKE ESTROGEN OR TO STOP TAKING IT AFTER MENOPAUSE?

A woman is advised not to take estrogen if she has or has had endometrial cancer. She may be advised not to take estrogen or to take it with extreme caution when she has or has had uterine abnormalities such as endometrial hyperplasia, fibroid tumors (myomas) of the uterus, uterine polyps, endometriosis, or adenomyosis. A woman taking estrogen who develops any of these diseases or conditions is usually advised to stop taking it because these conditions are believed to be estrogen dependent and may become worse when estrogen is taken.

DOES TAKING ESTROGEN WITHOUT PROGESTERONE OR PROGESTINS INCREASE A WOMAN'S RISK OF DEVELOPING UTERINE CANCER?

Continuous stimulation of the uterine lining (endometrium) by the estrogens estradiol and estrone has been shown to increase a woman's chances for developing uterine cancer.

Although estriol has been shown to be generally protective against the development of cancer in a woman's body after menopause, there is insufficient evidence to conclude that estriol alone is protective against uterine cancer when taken without natural progesterone or a progestin.

WHY WOULD A WOMAN TAKE ESTROGEN WITHOUT A PROGESTIN OR NATURAL PROGESTERONE?

Progestins are believed to increase a woman's risk for developing breast cancer and they appear to offset the benefits of estrogen on the cardiovascular system. Natural progesterone does not appear to have these disadvantages, although scientific double-blind studies have not been conducted to document its effectiveness.

Progestins and natural progesterone have also been known to cause a woman's menstrual periods to resume after menopause. Although they are usually lighter than premenopausal menstrual periods and diminish over time, many women find this a disagreeable side effect of taking a progestin or natural progesterone.

IS ALL POSTMENOPAUSAL BLEEDING THAT OCCURS WHILE A WOMAN IS TAKING HRT NORMAL?

Postmenopausal bleeding while a woman is taking *HRT* seriously concerns doctors because it can be a warning sign that the uterine lining (endometrium) is developing abnormalities that could lead to uterine cancer. Always report any bleeding you notice while taking *HRT* to your physician and discuss what tests you may need to ascertain if the bleeding is caused by uterine abnormalities.

HOW DOES A WOMAN'S DOCTOR DETERMINE THE CAUSE OF HER POSTMENOPAUSAL BLEEDING?

It is important to determine the origin of any abnormal bleeding a woman experiences at any time of her life, but especially during the perimenopausal years and after menopause, whether or not she takes *HRT.*

A pelvic exam will tell the doctor if your uterus feels abnormal or if the bleeding originates in your vagina. If that is not conclusive, a tampon can be useful in determining the source. The tampon is worn for a short period of time. If the bleeding continues and the tampon is free of blood when it is removed, the bleeding most likely comes from the bladder, urethra, or rectum area. A urologic evaluation may be suggested to discover whether the bleeding originates from the bladder, or a proctoscopic exam may be necessary to determine if the bleeding originates in the rectum.

WHAT TESTS CAN A DOCTOR CONDUCT TO DETERMINE THE CAUSE OF ABNORMAL BLEEDING THAT APPEARS TO COME FROM THE UTERUS?

If abnormal bleeding is believed to come from the uterus, various tests may be performed to determine its cause. These tests may be noninvasive, but a surgical procedure may be needed to acquire an endometrial tissue sample for analysis.

WHAT NONINVASIVE TESTS CAN DETERMINE THE CAUSE OF ABNORMAL UTERINE BLEEDING?

A vaginal ultrasound is sometimes used as a precautionary diagnostic evaluation for monitoring the thickness of a woman's uterine lining while she is taking *HRT.* Generally, if the uterine lining looks normal and the thickness of the endometrium is 5-mm or less, no further tests are warranted. If the endometrium is more than 5-mm thick, further tests are usually advised. Ultrasounds can also diagnose or monitor uterine fibroid tumors.

A medical D and C is hormonal therapy sometimes used if a woman has abnormal uterine bleeding. She takes progesterone pills for 7 to 14 days for one month to cause the uterine lining to shed once the progesterone is stopped, just as it would during a menstrual period. Sometimes this eliminates abnormal uterine bleeding caused by hormonal imbalances, however an endometrial tissue sample is unavailable for analysis that might identify a more serious cause for bleeding. If abnormal bleeding persists after a medical D and C, surgical evaluation may be recommended by your physician.

WHAT SURGICAL PROCEDURES MAY BE NEEDED TO DETERMINE THE CAUSE OF ABNORMAL UTERINE BLEEDING?

Various surgical procedures are used to determine the cause of abnormal uterine bleeding, including:

- an endometrial biopsy where a thin tube is inserted through the cervix into the uterus. An instrument scrapes the uterine lining and traps samples of tissue that are withdrawn along with the tube. This endometrial tissue sample is evaluated by a laboratory.

- aspiration of the uterine cavity is performed by inserting a thin tube through the cervix into the uterus. A syringe or suction machine attached to the tube suctions the uterine lining, removing more tissue than is taken for an endometrial biopsy. This tissue sample is also evaluated by a laboratory.

- surgical D and C (dilation and curettage) is performed by dilating the cervical opening, then inserting a spoon-shaped instrument into the uterus to scrape and remove as much of the uterine lining as necessary. These tissue samples are evaluated by a laboratory.

- hysteroscopy is performed by inserting a narrow light-containing telescope through the cervix into the uterus so the physician can look inside the uterus for abnormalities. A biopsy, aspiration, or D and C may then be performed if needed.

WHAT TYPES OF UTERINE ABNORMALITIES MIGHT BE FOUND DURING TESTS OF THESE KINDS?

These tests are usually performed to determine the cause for abnormal uterine bleeding, which may include endometrial hyperplasia, endometrial cancer, uterine polyps, endometriosis, adenomyosis, or fibroid tumors.

WHAT IS ENDOMETRIAL HYPERPLASIA?

Endometrial hyperplasia occurs when the glands and tissue of the uterine lining multiply, resulting in an abnormal number of glands that appear to be lying on top of each other rather than separated by supporting tissue. In severe cases (atypical endometrial hyperplasia), cells within the glands become irregular. Although this is usually benign cell development, it may be a warning sign that the development of endometrial cancer is possible.

HOW IS THAT DIFFERENT FROM ENDOMETRIAL CANCER?

In endometrial cancer the glands invade the supporting tissue around the uterus. If that invasion progresses, it can spread to other vital organs.

WHAT ARE THE SYMPTOMS OF ENDOMETRIAL HYPERPLASIA AND ENDOMETRIAL CANCER?

The most common sign of endometrial hyperplasia or endometrial cancer is abnormal uterine bleeding, which is why it is important to report any abnormal bleeding to your physician, especially when you take estrogen.

DOES TAKING ESTROGEN CAUSE ENDOMETRIAL HYPERPLASIA OR ENDOMETRIAL CANCER?

Cancer is not caused by taking estrogen, but excessive estrogen stimulation of the endometrial lining without progesterone is known to result in endometrial hyperplasia and can lead to endometrial cancer.

ARE ALL WOMEN AT EQUAL RISK FOR DEVELOPING ENDOMETRIAL HYPERPLASIA OR ENDOMETRIAL CANCER?

Any situation that causes the uterus to receive excessive estrogen stimulation without progesterone to counteract the uterine lining building-up is more prone to develop these diseases. That would include women who take estrogen during and after menopause without a progestin or natural progesterone.

Before menopause, a woman who does not ovulate regularly, especially if she has only a few menstrual periods a year, is at higher risk for developing endometrial hyperplasia or endometrial cancer. A woman who is very overweight is also at higher risk because her body fat converts androgens to estrogen.

HOW DOES A WOMAN KNOW IF ENDOMETRIAL HYPERPLASIA OR ENDOMETRIAL CANCER ARE CAUSING ABNORMAL BLEEDING?

Endometrial tissue samples will need to be taken and analyzed to determine if they are normal or appear to have the abnormal development associated with cancer.

WHAT ARE UTERINE POLYPS?

A uterine polyp is a growth that forms in the lining of the uterus, called an endometrial polyp, or in the endocervix, the canal leading

to the uterine cavity. Polyps form for various reasons, including excessive estrogen stimulation, and commonly occur during perimenopausal years when a woman's hormone production becomes
erratic. They may also develop from a small piece of pregnancy tissue left behind after childbirth, abortion, or miscarriage. There appears
to be a hereditary tendency to develop polyps.

ARE POLYPS CANCEROUS?

Uterine polyps are usually benign, especially during a woman's
thirties and forties, but the chances of their being malignant (cancerous) increase somewhat after menopause. Endocervical polyps
that develop before or after menopause are almost always benign.

HOW DOES A WOMAN KNOW IF POLYPS
ARE CAUSING HER ABNORMAL BLEEDING?

Either abnormal menstrual bleeding and spotting or very heavy
and prolonged periods can be a symptom of polyps. Your physician may be able to see endocervical polyps protruding from your
cervix during a pelvic exam, but uterine polyps hide within uterine tissue and can be confirmed only by more extensive endometrial examination, such as a D and C or a hysteroscopy.

WHAT IS ENDOMETRIOSIS?

Endometriosis is a disease caused by the uterine glands and tissue
migrating outside the uterine cavity and invading other pelvic areas.

HOW IS ENDOMETRIOSIS DIFFERENT FROM
ENDOMETRIAL HYPERPLASIA OR CANCER?

The configuration of the endometrial cells differs with each condition or disease.

HOW DOES A WOMAN KNOW IF
SHE HAS ENDOMETRIOSIS?

Endometriosis in perimenopausal women can cause severe menstrual cramps and painful periods, ovarian cysts, and can interfere with ovarian function. Endometriosis usually disappears after menopause when estrogen production by the ovaries diminishes.

WHAT IS ADENOMYOSIS?

Adenomyosis, also called internal endometriosis, occurs when the glands inside the uterine cavity grow into the muscle of the uterus.

HOW DOES A WOMAN KNOW IF SHE HAS ADENOMYOSIS?

Commonly found during the perimenopausal years when hormone production is imbalanced by excessive estrogen, adenomyosis may cause heavy bleeding and prolonged menstrual periods, with a feeling of heaviness in the abdomen. During a pelvic exam, a woman's doctor may find her uterus enlarged, soft and tender, but smooth (unlike the presence of fibroids, which cause the uterus to feel hard and lumpy).

WHAT ARE UTERINE FIBROID TUMORS?

A uterine fibroid (myoma or leiomyoma) is a benign growth of the uterine muscle that may be as small as a pea or as large as a basketball.

ARE ALL WOMEN AT EQUAL RISK FOR DEVELOPING UTERINE FIBROIDS?

About one of every four women over 30 has uterine fibroids, with black women having them more frequently.

HOW DOES A WOMAN KNOW IF UTERINE FIBROIDS ARE CAUSING ABNORMAL BLEEDING?

Smaller fibroids are usually painless and symptomless. Larger fibroids often can be felt through the abdominal cavity and may cause pain, pressure, and a feeling of heaviness in the abdomen. They may cause excessive uterine bleeding, constipation because of pressure on the rectum, and frequent urination due to pressure on the bladder.

Your doctor may suspect you have a uterine fibroid if your uterus feels hard, lumpy, enlarged, or irregularly shaped. Ultrasound may be recommended to confirm a uterine fibroid, as opposed to a more serious pelvic condition.

DO FIBROIDS TURN INTO UTERINE CANCER?

Uterine fibroids are benign and do not turn into cancer. They are usually not treated unless they grow large enough to cause pain or excessive menstrual bleeding. Because they are believed to be caused by excessive estrogen stimulation of the uterus, a woman with a uterine fibroid is usually advised not to take estrogen during and after menopause. Uterine fibroids often atrophy after menopause when a woman's natural production of estrogen drops off.

Some women with uterine fibroids may decide to take *HRT* for other health reasons (the benefits to their cardiovascular system or bones), but are extra cautious about the types and dosages of hormones they take and careful monitoring will be needed.

VAGINA CHANGES

DOES A WOMAN'S EXTERNAL GENITAL AREA CHANGE AFTER MENOPAUSE?

Diminished estrogen production by a woman's body as well as the normal aging process usually results in thinning of pubic hair and a wrinkling of her vulva, as her skin loses elasticity and some fat content. The labia may become less sensitive and less likely to swell and separate during sexual stimulation after years of lower estrogen production by the body.

WHAT CHANGES TAKE PLACE IN A WOMAN'S VAGINA AFTER MENOPAUSE?

Besides the vaginal dryness discussed in chapter 7, structural changes take place in the vagina after menopause when estrogen production within the body diminishes dramatically. Vaginal atrophy or postmenopausal vaginitis can occur after menopause because the vagina and surrounding tissues are among the most sensitive estrogen-dependent parts of a woman's body.

WHAT IS VAGINAL ATROPHY?

Before menopause, the estrogen-rich vaginal lining is normally several layers thick. Lack of estrogen during menopause causes the vaginal tissue to become thinner and more fragile, losing elasticity and lubricating capability, and causing it to change shape. This is called vaginal atrophy.

Before menopause, the vagina is normally two-and-a-half to-four inches long, with the cervix protruding into the vagina. After menopause, the vagina tends to constrict, becoming shorter and narrower close to the cervix, which tends to flatten. The vagina does not stretch as easily and is more prone to damage and bleeding when penetrated, which can result in uncomfortable sexual intercourse.

WHAT IS POSTMENOPAUSAL VAGINITIS?

After menopause, when the estrogen-deficient vaginal lining is reduced to only a few layers of cells, the vagina is more prone to infection. When it recurs, this condition is called postmenopausal vaginitis. It can cause a burning and itching feeling, sometimes accompanied by an unpleasant yellow or light green vaginal discharge, bleeding, or spotting.

IS VAGINAL BLEEDING AFTER MENOPAUSE ALWAYS CAUSED BY VAGINAL ATROPHY?

Vaginal bleeding is most commonly caused by vaginal atrophy, but it can also be a warning sign that something more serious is happening in your body. Therefore any vaginal bleeding after your menstrual periods have stopped needs to be reported to your physician so the cause can be determined, especially if you are taking *HRT.*

Vaginal bleeding can be confused with bleeding from the urinary bladder or urethra. Postmenopausal bleeding can be a warning sign that there are abnormalities of the uterine lining.

HOW SOON AFTER MENOPAUSE CAN VAGINAL ATROPHY OCCUR?

Every woman is different, but vaginal atrophy usually develops 3 to 10 years after menopause, with the average being 4 to 5 years after a woman's last menstrual period. However, some women experience vaginal dryness and painful intercourse even before their final menstrual period, and within three to six months after menopause caused by surgical removal of the ovaries.

DO ALL WOMEN DEVELOP VAGINAL ATROPHY AFTER MENOPAUSE?

Most women develop vaginal atrophy to some degree after menopause. The extent to which a woman's pelvic organs change after menopause depends on her individual genetic profile and her overall health and lifestyle. The functioning of a woman's endocrine glands affects her body's ability to make hormonal adjustments after her ovaries stop producing hormones.

DOES TAKING ESTROGEN PREVENT A WOMAN FROM DEVELOPING VAGINAL ATROPHY?

Because vaginal atrophy is directly related to the body's production of estrogen, taking estrogen after menopause has been shown to significantly decrease a woman's chances of developing vaginal atrophy.

Some foods, supplements, and herbs also have an estrogen effect on the body and those discussed in chapter 6 may be useful for keeping your pelvic organs toned by maintaining tissue elasticity during and after menopause.

HOW DOES A WOMAN KNOW IF SHE'S DEVELOPING VAGINAL ATROPHY?

Vaginal dryness and painful intercourse are usually the first signs of vaginal atrophy. Frequent vaginal bleeding after intercourse, persistent vaginal irritation, or infections need to be reported to your physician.

CAN A WOMAN'S DOCTOR TELL IF SHE'S DEVELOPING VAGINAL ATROPHY?

During a pelvic exam your physician may detect the following signs of vaginal atrophy: an estrogen-rich vaginal lining will be pink, thick, well lubricated, with many folds, as opposed to looking pale, thin, dry, and flattened after vaginal atrophy has developed. A maturation index can also be done to determine estrogen effect on the vagina.

WHAT IS A MATURATION INDEX?

A maturation index is also called an estrogen index. It is performed by scraping cells from the vaginal wall in the same way a Pap smear is taken from the cervix. These vaginal cells are examined under a microscope to determine the numbers of three types of cells normally present in the vagina: superficial cells, parabasal cells, and basal cells. The percentage of these three different types of cells reveals estrogen effect on the vaginal lining.

There are three sets of numbers in a maturation index, one for each type of cell. A larger proportion of superficial cells indicates a strong estrogen effect in the vagina, while an absence of them indicates lack of estrogen, usually as a result of menopause.

HOW CAN A WOMAN INTERPRET HER MATURATION INDEX?

The three numbers in a maturation index will be reported in this manner: 100-0-0 or 0-60-40. The first number is basal cells, the second parabasal, the third superficial.

When a woman menstruates regularly there is usually significant estrogen effect on the vagina and the maturation index may read something like 0-40-60. As estrogen decreases after menopause the index may become something like 5-90-5. An absence of estrogen effect on the vagina will show up in a maturation index as 100-0-0.

While a woman is still menstruating the maturation index will change slightly during her menstrual cycle.

DOES THE MATURATION INDEX TELL A WOMAN'S DOCTOR IF SHE NEEDS TO TAKE HRT DURING AND AFTER MENOPAUSE?

Although hormone production by the ovaries influences the entire body, the maturation index is used only to determine estrogen effect on the vagina. It is not considered a reliable gauge of estrogen effects on the cardiovascular system or the bones of a woman. Other tests for determining a woman's overall need for HRT are described in chapter 3.

DOES HRT ELIMINATE POSTMENOPAUSAL VAGINITIS?

Taking estrogen eliminates postmenopausal vaginitis in most women after menopause.

Antibiotics may be needed to treat vaginal inflammation and infection caused by lack of estrogen, but with recurring vaginitis a woman may need to take estrogen to reestablish vaginal mucus and increase the thickness of her vaginal tissue.

CAN ESTROGEN CREAM USED VAGINALLY HELP PREVENT VAGINAL ATROPHY AND POSTMENOPAUSAL VAGINITIS?

Estrogen cream inserted vaginally has been shown to be very helpful in treating vaginal atrophy and vaginitis. It improves lubrication and enhances the thickness of vaginal tissue when used a few times a week.

However, estrogen applied vaginally still gets absorbed into a woman's general circulation, although the rate of absorption is not as predictable as other types of estrogen intake.

IS IT SAFE FOR A WOMAN TO USE A SMALL AMOUNT OF ESTROGEN CREAM VAGINALLY IF SHE CANNOT TAKE ESTROGEN ORALLY?

A woman who cannot take estrogen orally needs to discuss with her physician whether it is safe for her to insert small amounts of estrogen cream vaginally to prevent vaginal atrophy or vaginitis. All health factors need to be considered and close monitoring may be needed, especially if irregular bleeding or other symptoms occur in conjunction with estrogen cream use.

WHAT CAN A WOMAN DO TO PREVENT VAGINAL ATROPHY AND VAGINITIS IF SHE CANNOT TAKE HRT?

Regular sexual intercourse is said to help keep a woman's vagina from becoming shorter as her estrogen levels start dropping. A woman who is not sexually active can dilate her vagina with her fingers a few times a week, using a water-soluble lubricant to avoid irritation to the thinning vaginal tissue. Medical supply companies sell vaginal dilators for women who are not comfortable using their fingers.

Vaginal lubricants effectively eliminate vaginal dryness, reduce vaginal irritation during intercourse, and reduce the incidence of vaginitis. Water-soluble lubricants are best. Avoid lubricants that contain perfumes or chemicals, as well as petroleum-based lubricants (such as petroleum jelly and mineral oils), because they may irritate the delicate vaginal lining and increase your risk of developing vaginitis.

Vitamin E vaginal suppositories or a few drops of vitamin E liquid inserted into the vagina a few times a week have also been known to be an effective alternative to estrogen.

IS THERE ANYTHING A WOMAN CAN DO TO AVOID TAKING ANTIBIOTICS FOR VAGINITIS?

Folk remedies have been used for centuries in treating yeastlike inflammations and irritations of the vagina. They include yogurt (with active culture) douches, eating yogurt or garlic, and taking acidophilus capsules daily, while avoiding sugar, including very sweet fruit.

Practical tips for avoiding and arresting vaginal irritation include avoiding tight-fitting clothing that does not allow for air circulation in the vaginal area, avoiding panties and pantyhose with dyes that may be irritating, and avoiding laundry detergents and fabric softeners that can irritate delicate vaginal tissue.

If you have to take antibiotics, they will destroy the beneficial bacteria in the body and recurrence of the condition may result, as well as possible urinary tract or bladder irritation or infection. You can reestablish your body's beneficial bacteria by eating yogurt with active cultures or by taking acidophilus.

Conclusion

Every woman's healthcare needs are different, with various factors determining whether she feels safe and comfortable with her healthcare choices. It is important for your doctor to do more than dispense medications to treat your symptoms or a disease. Healthcare during menopause also involves providing information about any medications you choose to take, offering suggestions about your diet and nutritional intake, as well as lifestyle changes and supplements that may enhance your overall health, based on your personal health profile.

Although conventional medical treatment is often the first choice of Americans, a recent national poll revealed that one of three Americans is now incorporating natural or alternative healthcare into their health maintenance programs along with conventional medicine.

Selecting healthcare support, assistance, and guidance that is effective and comfortable may be the biggest challenge for a woman today. Although there are many choices and options, most women don't know where to find the help they want. The Suggested Reading List and Resources appendices, and the Sources may help you obtain more information on the specific healthcare programs that interest you.

Suggested
Reading List

Ford, Gillian. *What's Wrong with My Hormones?* Newcastle, CA: Desmond Ford Publications, 1992.

Futterman, Lori, R.N., Ph.D., and Jones, John E., Ph.D. *The PMS and Perimenopause Sourcebook.* Los Angeles: Lowell House, 1997.

Gaby, Alan R., M.D. *Preventing and Reversing Osteoporosis.* Prima Publishing, Box 1260BK, Rocklin, CA 95677, 916-786-0426. Published 1993.
Discusses natural progesterone and estriol, as well as nutrition for treating and preventing osteoporosis and other women's health concerns

Gittleman, Ann Louise. *Super Nutrition for Menopause.* New York: Pocket Books, 1993.

Henkel Gretchen. *Making the Estrogen Decision.* Los Angeles: Lowell House, 1992.

Henkel, Gretchen. *The Menopause Sourcebook.* Los Angeles: Lowell House, 1996.

Kamen, Betty. *Hormone Replacement Therapy: Yes or No?* Nutrition Encounter, Inc., Box 5847, Novato, CA 94948. Published 1993.
Discusses natural progesterone and nutrition for the treatment of women's health during and after menopause

Lee, John, M.D. *What Your Doctor May Not Tell You About Menopause.* Available through the Allergy Resources Catalog, 1-800-USE-FLAX.

Lee, John R., M.D. *Natural Progesterone, The Multiple Roles of a Remarkable Hormone.* BLL Publishing, Box 2068, Sebastapol, CA, 95473. Published 1993.
Discusses natural progesterone in women's healthcare

Ryneveld, Edna Copeland. *Secrets of a Natural Menopause, A Positive Drug-Free Approach.* St. Paul, MN: Llewellyn Publications, 1995.

Stewart, Felicia, M.D., Guest, Felicia, Stewart, Gary, M.D., and Hatcher, Robert, M.D. *My Body, My Health: The Concerned Woman's Guide to Gynecology.* New York: John Wiley and Sons, 1979

Stoppard, Miriam. *Menopause: The Complete Practical Guide to Managing Your Life and Maintaining Physical and Emotional Well-Being.* New York: Dorling Kindersley Publishing, Inc., 1994.

Resources for Information, Products, and Practitioners

Natural progesterone

Bezwecken Transdermal
Beaverton, OR
503-644-7800

Professional and Technical Services, Inc.
Portland, OR
503-226-1010 or 800 648-8211

Natural progesterone, estriol, and referrals to physicians familiar with natural hormones:

ApotheCure
Dallas, TX
1-800-969-6601

College Pharmacy
Colorado Springs, CO
1-800-888-9358

Women's International Pharmacy
5708 Monona Drive
Madison, WI
608-221-7800 or 1-800 279-5708

Acupressure

Reed, Michael. *Acupressure's Potent Points: A Guide to Self-Care for Common Ailments.* New York: Bantam Books, 1990.

Acupuncture

American Academy of Medical Acupuncture
2520 Milvia Street
Berkeley, CA 94704
415-841-3220

American Association of Acupuncture & Oriental Medicine
4104 Lake Boone Trail, Suite 201
Raleigh, NC 27607
919-787-5181

Aromatherapy

Rose, Jeanne. *The Aromatherapy Book: Applications and Inhalations.*
Berkeley, CA: North Atlantic Books, 1992.

Walji, Hasnain. *The Healing Power of Aromatherapy.* Rocklin, CA:
Prima Publishing, 1996.

Ayurvedic Medicine

Maharishi Ayurveda Health Center for Stress Management and
Behavioral Medicine
679 Gorge Hill Road
P.O. Box 344
Lancaster, MA 01523
508-365-4549

Biofeedback

American Association of Biofeedback Clinicians
2424 Dempster
Des Plaines, IL 60016
312-827-0440

Cardiovascular

American Heart Association
7310 Greenville Avenue
Dallas, TX 75231
1-800-AHA-8721
Referrals and literature available

Arizona Heart Institute and Foundation
2632 North 20th Street
Phoenix, AZ 85006
602-266-2200
Informational brochures available

Chinese Herbalism

American College of Traditional Chinese Medicine
455 Arkansas Street
San Francisco, CA 94107
415-282-7600 or 415-282-9603

Health Concerns
8001 Capwell Drive
Oakland, CA 94621
510-639-0280

Hsu, Hong Yen. *For Women Only: Chinese Herbal Formulas*
Available through the Allergy Resources Catalog, 1-800-USE-FLAX.

Chiropractic

American Chiropractic Association
1916 Wilson Boulevard
Arlington, VA 22201
703-276-8800

World Chiropractic Alliance
2950 N. Dobson Road
Chandler, AZ 85224
1-800-347-1011

Herbalism

Brown, Donald J. *Herbal Prescriptions for Better Health*. Rocklin, CA:
Prima Publishing, 1996.

Castleman, Michael. *The Healing Herbs*. Emmaus, PA: Rodale Press, 1991.

Murray, Michael. *The Healing Power of Herbs*. Rocklin, CA: Prima
Publishing, 1996

Headache

National Headache Foundation
4242 North Western Avenue
Chicago, IL 60625
1-800-843-2256

Holistic Medicine

American Holistic Medical Association
2002 East Lake Avenue East
Seattle, WA 98101
206-322-6842

Homeopathy

International Foundation for Homeopathy
P.O. Box 7
Edmonds, WA 98020
206-776-4147

National Center for Homeopathy
801 North Fairfax Street, Suite 306
Alexandria, VA 22314
703-548-7790

Cummings, Stephen and Ullman, Dana. *Everybody's Guide to Homeopathic Medicines.* Los Angeles: J.P. Tarcher, 1991.

Grossinger, Richard. *Homeopathy: An Introduction for Skeptics and Beginners.* Berkeley, CA: North Atlantic Books, 1992.

Homeopathic Medicine for Women. Available through the Allergy Resources Catalog, 1-800-USE-FLAX.

Menopause

As We Change, catalogue of menopause related products
1-800-203-5585

North American Menopause Society
University Hospitals
Department of Obstetrics and Gynecology
11100 Euclid Avenue
Cleveland, OH 44106
216-844-3334
Will provide a list of healthcare practitioners who specialize in the treatment of menopause

Naturopathy

American Association of Naturopathic Physicians
2366 Eastlake Avenue East, Suite 322
Seattle, WA 98102

Obstetrics and Gynecology

American College of Obstetricians and Gynecologists (ACOG)
Resource Center
409 12th Street, SW
Washington, DC 20024-2188
202-638-5577
Send SASE for pamphlet AP047, "The Menopause Years"

Osteoporosis

National Osteoporosis Center
1150 17th Street, NW, Suite 500
Washington, DC 20036-4603
202-223-2226
Informational pamphlets available

Calcium w/Out The Cou. Available through the Allergy Resources
Catalog, 1800-USE-FLAX.

Stress Reduction

American Institute of Stress
124 Park Avenue
Yonkers, NY 10703
914-963-1200 or 1-800-24-RELAX

International Stress Management Association
10455 Pomerado Road
San Diego, CA 92131
619-693-4698

Visualization

Mind/Body Health Sciences, Inc.
393 Dixon Road
Boulder, CO 80302
303-440-8460

Women's Health

A Friend Indeed Publications, Inc.
P.O. Box 1710
Champlain, NY 12919-1710
Menopause related newsletter for subscription fee. Free first
issue with SASE

Menopause News
2074 Union Street
San Francisco, CA 94123
Newsletter for subscription fee. Free first issue with SASE

National Women's Health Network
514 10th Street, NW, Suite 400
Washington, DC 20004
202-347-1140
Provides referrals and literature

Women's Health Letter
P.O. Box 467939
Atlanta, GA 31146-7939
770-399-5617 or 1-800-728-2288
Monthly newsletter available for subscription fee

Yoga

Yoga Journal
2054 University Avenue, Suite 601
Berkeley, CA 94704-1082
Magazine available at newstands. Lists classes and workshops nationwide

References

The information in this book was compiled from sources selected because of the extensive medical documentation they provide. You may want to review these sources or read the actual medical reports referred to in the following books or publications. Medical reports referenced in these sources may be obtained at medical libraries and in some public libraries.

Altman, Nat, *Everybody's Guide to Chiropractic Health Care.* Los Angeles, CA: J.P. Tarcher, 1990.

Budoff, Penny Wise, M.D., *No More Hot Flashes and Other Good News.* New York: Warner Books, 1989.

Cutler, Winnifred B., and C-R. Garcia, *Menopause: A Guide for Women and the Men Who Love Them.* New York: W.W. Norton and Co., 1992.

Doress, Paula B., and Diane L. Siegal, Mid-Life and Older Women's Book Project (editors), *Ourselves Growing Older.* New York: Simon and Schuster, 1987.

Follingstad, A.H., "Estriol, the forgotten estrogen?" *Journal of American Medical Association,* January 2, 1978, 239:29–30.

Ford, Gillian, *What's Wrong with My Hormones?* Newcastle, CA: D. Ford Publications, 1992.

Frisch, Melvin, M.D., *Stay Cool Through Menopause.* New York: The Body Press/Perigee Books, 1993.

Gaby, Alan R., M.D., *Preventing and Reversing Osteoporosis.* Rocklin, CA: Prima Publishing, 1994.

Gittleman, Ann Louise, *Super Nutrition for Menopause.* New York: Pocket Books, 1993.

Greenwood, Sadja. *Menopause Naturally: Preparing for the Second Half of Life*. Volcano, CA: Volcano Press, 1992.

Harvard Women's Health Watch. Boston, MA: monthly newsletter.

Henkel, Gretchen, *Making the Estrogen Decision*. Los Angeles, CA: Lowell House, 1992.

Kamen, Betty, Ph.D., *Hormone Replacement Therapy, Yes or No?* Novato, CA: Nutrition Encounter, Inc., 1993.

Kastner, Mark, and Hugh Burroughs, *Alternative Healing: The Complete A–Z Guide to Over 160 Different Alternative Therapies*. Halcyon, CA: Halcyon Book Concern, 1993.

Lad, Vasant, *Ayurveda: The Science of Self-Healing. A Practical Guide*. Santa Fe, NM: Lotus Press, 1985.

Lavabre, Marcel F., *Aromatherapy Workbook*. Rochester, VT: Healing Arts Press, 1990.

Lee, John R., M.D., *Natural Progesterone*. Sebastopol, CA: BLL Publishing, 1993.

Lemon, H.M., "Reduced estriol excretion in patients with breast cancer prior to endocrine therapy," *Journal of American Medical Association*. 1966, 196:112–120.

Lockie, Andrew, *The Women's Guide to Homeopathy: The Natural Way to a Healthier Life for Women*. New York: St. Martins Press, 1994.

McCain, Marian Van Eyk, *Transformation Through Menopause*. New York: Bergen and Garvey, 1991.

Mindell, Earl, *Vitamin Bible*. New York: Warner Books.

Murray, M.T., *The Healing Power of Herbs*. Rocklin, CA: Prima Publishing, 1992.

Nissim, Rina, *Natural Healing in Gynecology*. New York: Pandora Press, 1986.

Perry, Susan, and Katherine O'Hanlan, M.D., *Natural Menopause: The Complete Guide to a Woman's Most Misunderstood Passage*. New York: Addison-Wesley, 1992.

Reitz, Rosetta. *Menopause—A Positive Approach*. New York: Random House, 1992.

Salaman, Maureen, *Foods That Heal.* Menlo Park, CA: MKS, Inc., 1994.

Smith, Trevor, M.D., *Homeopathic Medicine for Women, An Alternative Approach to Gynecological Health Care.* Rochester, VT: Healing Arts Press.

Stein, Diane, *The Natural Remedy Book for Women.* Freedom, CA: Crossing Press, 1992.

Stewart, Felicia, M.D., Felicia Guest, Gary Stewart, M.D., and Robert Hatcher, M.D., *My Body, My Health: The Concerned Woman's Guide to Gynecology.* New York: John Wiley and Sons, 1979.

Utian, Wulf H., and Ruth Jacobowitz, *Managing Your Menopause.* New York: Simon and Schuster/Fireside Press, 1992.

Wagner, Edward M., M.D., and Sylvia Goldfarb, *How to Stay Out of The Doctor's Office: An Encyclopedia For Alternative Healing.* New York: Instant Improvement, Inc., 1992.

Weil, Andrew, *Health and Healing: Understanding Conventional and Alternative Medicine.* Boston: Houghton Mifflin, 1983.

Whitaker, Julian, M.D. *Health and Healing.* Potomac, MD: monthly newsletter.

Index